40 DAYS TO
BETTER
LIVING

HYPERTENSION

BARBOUR
PUBLISHING

Published by Barbour Publishing, Inc., P.O. Box 719, Uhrichsville,
Ohio 44683, www.barbourbooks.com

*Our mission is to publish and distribute inspirational products
offering exceptional value and biblical encouragement to the
masses.*

Member of the
Evangelical Christian
Publishers Association

Printed in the United States of America.

TABLE OF CONTENTS

Welcome,
from Dr. Scott Morris,
Founder of the Church Health Center

I first came to Memphis in 1986. I had no personal ties to Memphis and did not know anyone here. Having completed theological and medical education, I was determined to begin a health care ministry for the working poor. The next year, the doors of the Church Health Center opened with one doctor—me—and one nurse. We saw twelve patients the first day. Today we handle about 36,000 patient visits a year and 120,000 visits to our Wellness facility. A staff of 250 people shares a ministry of healing and wellness while hundreds more volunteer time and services.

So what sets us apart from other community clinics around the country?

The Church Health Center is fundamentally about the Church. We care for our patients without relying on government funds because God calls the Church to healing work. Jesus' life was about healing the whole person—body and spirit—and the Church is Jesus in the world. His message is our message. His ministry is our ministry. Local congregations embrace this calling and help make our work possible.

More than two decades of caring for the working uninsured makes one thing plain: health care needs to change. In the years that the Church Health Center has cared for people in Memphis, we've seen that two-thirds of our patients seek treatment for illness that healthier living can prevent or control. We realize that if we want to make a lasting difference in our patients' lives, the most effective strategy is encouraging overall wellness in body and spirit. At a fundamental level, we must transform what the words *well* and *health* mean in the minds of most people.

To do that, we developed the Model for Healthy Living. Living healthy lives doesn't just mean that you see the doctor regularly. Rather, healthy living means that all aspects of your life are in balance. Your faith, work, nutrition, movement, family and friends, emotions, and medical health all contribute to a life filled with more joy, more love, and more connection to God.

How to Use This Book

This book provides opportunities to improve your health in whatever way you need to for your optimal wellness. For the next forty days, we invite you to be inspired by the real-life people whose lives have been changed by the Church Health Center. Each day offers us a new chance to improve our health, so each day we will give you helpful ways that you can make your life healthier.

Some days you may choose to focus on just one or two of our "tips": Faith Life, Medical, Movement, Work, Emotional, Family and Friends, or Nutrition. Some days you may want to try all of them. The important thing is to remember that God calls us to an abundant life, and we can always make changes to strive for better health as it relates to hypertension.

Forty days and numerous ways to live a healthy life—come and join us on the journey!

Linda's Story

Linda came to the Church Health Center to begin an exercise program, as well as to use the clinic services. She knew she had hypertension, but had run out of her medication. When a clinic provider checked her blood pressure, it was much higher than anyone had expected, including Linda. That would have been a perfect time to give up, but she did not.

Now she is getting back on track. She sees a clinic provider to have her blood pressure monitored each time she comes into the Church Health Center. She is getting her medication filled on time so that she doesn't go back to where she was before she came to the Church Health Center. She started an extensive exercise program to get her body functioning as it should, sees a registered dietitian, and attends a hypertension education class.

Linda has a long way to go, but she has support aplenty at the Church Health Center. She knows where she is beginning, and she can start looking forward to the finish line. Both Linda and the team she is working with hope that in the next few months she can reduce the number of medications she must take and possibly even eliminate medication from her routine altogether.

She knows where she is beginning, and she can start looking forward to the finish line.

Day 1:
STARTING OUT

Morning Reflection

When Linda came into the Church Health Center, she was not aware of the severity of her condition. Hypertension symptoms might not show up until the hypertension is quite advanced, so by the time we are aware of a problem, it may seem insurmountable. But the way to move forward is to know exactly where you are beginning. Today, as we start out toward the goal, we will begin by planting our feet firmly on the starting line.

Faith Life
If you do not have a journal already, start one today. Take a few minutes and write ten words that describe your faith life right now. Be honest, and try to include both positive and negative aspects of your faith life.

Medical
Make a list of your medical concerns. Hypertension is among them, but hypertension often accompanies other medical issues. Having a list of your medical concerns will help you to set goals in the coming weeks and make your doctor's appointments more productive.

Movement

We all have to start somewhere. Go for a walk today, walking as far as you can. Do not exhaust yourself; stop when you feel you need to. Make a note in your journal so that you can track your progress.

Work

Work can be many things—your job, volunteering, hobbies, gardening, parenting. Make a list today of the many things that make up your "work." As you move forward on this journey, finding how to make healthy choices while you work will be important.

Emotional

As you set out on this journey, remember that emotional wellness is a crucial part of overall wellness. Today, take five minutes and write about your feelings as you begin this journey. What do you feel? Excitement? Fear? Nervousness?

Family and Friends

On this journey, support from family and friends will become very important. Take five minutes today and write the names of the family and friends who will support you on your destination to health.

Nutrition

Start a food journal, or add "food journaling" to your already current journal. Record what you eat today, including snacks and all meals. This will help you as you set your nutritional goals in the weeks to come.

Evening Wrap-Up

In the beginning you laid the foundations of the earth, and the heavens are the work of your hands.
PSALM 102:25

Congratulations! You have started your journey and made it through your first day! The beginning can be an especially difficult part of the task, and since this journey is the beginning of a new foundation, it can be even more difficult than we anticipate. But this is a journey about laying down a foundation for a new life. While that may seem impossible today, on Day One, we can call to mind the words of the psalmist: God "laid the foundations of the earth." If God laid the foundations of the earth, surely God walks with us as we lay the foundation to a healthier life. We can find encouragement and courage as we move forward on the journey.

Almighty God, help me today to find encouragement to lay a new foundation for my life. Help me to see You at work in my life as I set out on the journey toward wellness. In Your holy name, Amen.

Day 2:
Motivation

Morning Reflection

We all have different reasons for starting out on a journey. Wanting to live a wellness-oriented life can be a motivation in and of itself. Often, however, our motivation involves more than just wanting to feel healthier. Maybe we want to be able to play more with our kids. Maybe we simply want to stop taking so many medications. Whatever the motivation, it is important to know it and remember it as we set out on the journey, because it is this motivation that will keep us going.

Faith Life
Take five minutes and write in your journal about your spiritual motivation for being on this wellness journey. Is God with you on this journey? How is God involved?

Medical
If your motivation is medical, write down your medical motivation for this journey. Be as specific as possible. For example, if you would like to lower your blood pressure, write down the specific number that you have in mind.

Movement
After you take a shower (so that your muscles are

warm), spend five to ten minutes doing some light stretching. Bend and touch your toes. Reach your arms across your chest. (Hint: If it hurts, stop the stretch. You could tear a muscle if you push yourself too hard.)

Work

Sometimes our lack of wellness can keep us from doing the kind of work that we want to do. Take five minutes and write about a time when you found yourself unable to do the work you needed to accomplish. (Keep in mind that work can be career-oriented, but it does not need to be.)

Emotional

Deep breathing can help you to get centered, release stress, and gain energy. Take five minutes today and take some deep breaths. Close your eyes, take a deep breath in through your nose, and breathe out through your mouth.

Family and Friends

Family dinners are a wonderful way to connect with your family and friends. They are also a wonderful time to try new recipes. Today, schedule a family dinner for sometime in the next week, and try a new healthy recipe.

Nutrition

Most of us have a standard grocery list. What is yours? Take a few minutes today to write up a standard list of the food that you generally buy each week.

Evening Wrap-Up

Then God said, "Let us make mankind in our image, in our likeness." . . .So God created mankind in his own image, in the image of God he created them; male and female he created them. . .and it was very good.
GENESIS 1:26–27, 31

We are created in God's image. That is, our bodies are created in the image of God. But we can find it difficult to love our bodies (a part of God's creation) the way that God loves us. Part of this journey is learning to see ourselves as God sees us—as very good. We can trust that God loves His creation. God loves us. God calls us *very good*.

Lord God, help me to see myself in You.
On my journey toward wellness, help me to see myself as You see me—with love, and as a part of Your creation.
In Your holy name, Amen.

Day 3:
Setting Goals

Morning Reflection

This journey is about wellness and making changes. Linda was able to make a direct change in her life by getting back on track and committing to treating her hypertension. But undirected change will only leave us feeling overwhelmed or frantic. Setting realistic and smart goals is very important to making lasting lifestyle changes. In particular, effective goal-setting can help us to stay focused at those times when we meet barriers and are close to giving up. Today, we will turn our focus to setting healthy and realistic goals to overcome the barriers set before us.

Faith Life
Take five minutes today and write down one practical and concrete goal for the next six weeks. For example, set a goal that you will pray once a day each day at a particular time. The more specific and concrete the goal, the easier it will be to achieve.

Medical
Weight loss is often a medical goal that people set. If this is your goal, try to aim for one to two pounds per week. While weight loss can certainly be a part of a wellness-oriented lifestyle, it is not healthy to lose weight too rapidly.

Movement

Today write down three goals related to exercise, and place those goals in a spot where you will see them often. For example: Be able to walk for ten minutes without taking a break. Do ten wall push-ups. Do ten sit-ups.

Work

Return to the list you made two days ago of things that make up your work. What would you like to change about your work? What do you have the power and authority to change in your work?

Emotional

Hypertension can be exacerbated (and sometimes even caused) by stress. Today, write down a specific and concrete goal for managing your stress. Remember to set a definitive time frame for your goals.

Family and Friends

Are you embarking on this journey on your own or with a friend or some family members? Having a companion going through the same journey can be very helpful. Think today about a friend or family member whom you might reach out to.

Nutrition

What would you like to change about your nutritional habits? Consume less fat? Eat more vegetables? Choose better portion sizes? Write down five nutritional goals for the next six weeks.

Evening Wrap-Up

*Forgetting what is behind and straining toward
what is ahead, I press on toward the goal to win
the prize for which God has called me
heavenward in Christ Jesus.*
PHILIPPIANS 3:13–14

We are setting out on a journey both of physical
training and of spiritual training. Wellness is about
our bodies and our spirits. When we neglect one
in favor of the other, we forget that God created
us as body *and* spirit. As Paul writes in his first
letter to Timothy, our hope in God can offer us
encouragement and purpose as we strive toward
our goal.

*God of hope, help me to focus today. I pray that You would
help me strive for my goal as I care for this wonderful body
that You have given me. In Your holy name, Amen.*

Day 4:
Expectations

Morning Reflection

Halfway through the first week, this journey can already feel overwhelming. We are working to change deeply entrenched habits, and so, in many ways, we are swimming against the tide. But we can certainly get in the way of change when we hold ourselves and God to unrealistic expectations. Our expectations shape our day-to-day experience of wellness and of faith. Today, we will focus on what we expect of ourselves and God as we continue on this journey.

Faith Life
We all have expectations of God in our lives. What are your expectations of God on this journey? Take five minutes today and write about your expectations of God.

Medical
When making changes to our health, it is always important to consult professionals. Today, investigate whether a dietitian or other specialist can help you along this journey.

Movement
Spend ten minutes stretching today (after a walk or a hot shower so that your muscles are loose).

Can you stretch any farther than you did a couple of days ago? What are your expectations for a couple of days from now?

Work
When you take a break at work, what do you usually do? Take a trip to a vending machine? Grab a cup of coffee? Today, try going for a short walk instead of eating during your break.

Emotional
If we have unrealistic expectations for ourselves, then our stress level will increase, rather than become more manageable. Take five minutes and write, as honestly as you can, what your expectations are for the next six weeks and whether they are realistic or not.

Family and Friends
Sometimes we can feel that our family and friends have particular expectations of us, and that can add to the stress we are already feeling. Today, talk to a friend or family member about your journey and what your expectations include.

Nutrition
Our nutritional habits will not change overnight—nor will our tastes! Today, make a list of your favorite foods. Are they healthy foods? Comfort foods? Over the next six weeks, we can work on finding more nutritional ways to enjoy your favorite foods.

Evening Wrap-Up

*Even when I am old and gray, do not forsake me,
my God, till I declare your power to the next
generation, your mighty acts to all who are to
come. Your righteousness, God, reaches to the
heavens, you who have done great things.
Who is like you, God? Though you have made me
see troubles, many and bitter, you will restore
my life again; from the depths of the earth
you will again bring me up.*
PSALM 71:18–20

We all have expectations—good and bad. Sometimes our expectations may be unrealistic, and we can become discouraged. But whatever our expectations are, they are nothing compared to God's reality. God's power reaches the high heavens, and God cares for us, even when we are discouraged and feeling low. God's love is stronger than any expectations that we might have for ourselves.

Loving God, "from the depths of the earth you will again bring me up." Give me the encouragement and wisdom to continue on this journey to wellness. In Your holy name, Amen.

Day 5:
First Steps

Morning Reflection

Hypertension does not happen overnight, and neither does it disappear overnight. When we put one foot in front of the other, we can gradually gain some control over the symptoms and habits that brought us to hypertension in the first place. As with climbing any mountain, we must take our first steps well before we reach the summit. Today we will focus on taking those first steps toward managing hypertension.

Faith Life

First steps can be very intimidating. Today, read the story of Moses' initiation in Exodus 3. Notice that Moses tried lots of excuses to get out of the journey that God called him to take. Are there any parallels in Moses' story to your own journey?

Medical

Medical setbacks, such as learning about hypertension, can be devastating. Such setbacks need not be the end of the world, nor should they be cause to give up. Today, write out a plan for dealing with medical setbacks to discuss when you next meet with your primary care provider.

Movement

On Day 1 you went for a walk. Go for another walk

today and try to push yourself to walk a little farther. Again, do not exhaust yourself, but remember that you cannot grow if you do not step outside of your current limits.

Work
Instead of drinking coffee or soda at work today, try to drink water. Drinking plenty of water and staying hydrated will help your body work better, and cutting back on caffeine is certainly a first step toward managing your hypertension.

Emotional
Today, take five minutes and write about taking first steps. How are you feeling about your first steps this week? Proud? Intimidated? Frustrated? Getting your feelings down on paper is a great first step toward emotional wellness and stress management.

Family and Friends
What kind of support do you need from your family and friends? Take a few minutes to identify the kind of support that would be most helpful from your personal relationships, and then talk to a friend or family member about it.

Nutrition
Managing hypertension means cutting back on certain items in your diet, particularly cholesterol and sodium. Today, go to your pantry and read the labels on ten food items, taking special note of how much sodium is in each item.

Evening Wrap-Up

The poor and needy search for water, but there is none; their tongues are parched with thirst. But I the Lord will answer them; I, the God of Israel, will not forsake them. I will make rivers flow on barren heights, and springs within the valleys. I will turn the desert into pools of water, and the parched ground into springs.
Isaiah 41:17–18

First steps are sometimes the most difficult. It can feel fruitless as we take one measly step while we look up at the summit of the mountain, knowing just how far we have to go. But as we put one foot in front of the other, we can take refuge in the knowledge that God walks with us. This is the God who brings water from the desert. God tells us, "I, the God of Israel, will not forsake them."

Lord God, *walk with me as I take my first steps toward wellness. Help me to see Your hand moving in my life.* In Your holy name, Amen.

Day 6:
Setbacks

Morning Reflection

Linda knew that she had hypertension, but she was having trouble dealing with it until she came to the Church Health Center. As we gain some momentum on this journey, we must take a moment to recognize that setbacks can and do happen. Making true progress involves a lot of moving forward and then dealing with setbacks. True progress is slow and is measured over a long time, rather than by one day or one meal. But those setbacks, when we have them, can provide us an excuse to give up. Today, we will focus on how we can deal with setbacks when they inevitably arrive.

Faith Life
Think of a time in your faith life when you experienced a setback. Spend five minutes writing about that time. How did you move past it? Did you talk to a friend? Did you tell your pastor? Did you spend more time reading the Bible and praying?

Medical
If you do not know how to find your pulse, today is the day to learn! Use your index and middle fingers to feel your pulse at your wrist, below your thumb. Count the beats that you feel in fifteen seconds, and multiply the number by four. That is your standing heart rate.

Movement

Walk around your home, taking two steps forward and then one step backward. Notice how you still make forward progress, even when every third step is a step back.

Work

Work is a place where many of us have setbacks. Stress and time constraints make it easy to fall back into old (and bad) habits, such as vending machine lunches and caffeinated, sugary sodas. Today, try bringing a stress ball or some Silly Putty to your workplace to relieve stress.

Emotional

Many of us are "programmed" to assign more value to our setbacks than to our successes. Make a list of successes or small victories that you experienced today. For example, "I drank water instead of soda with my lunch." Celebrate those successes!

Family and Friends

When you have a setback, your family and friends can help remind you of your successes. Today, name two people you can count on to offer encouragement and perspective in the event of a setback.

Nutrition

Nutritional setbacks happen. We have an occasional donut or eat a little more than we had intended at a dinner out. Though the temptation is to starve ourselves the next day, the better way to deal with those setbacks is to simply get back to healthy, moderate eating the next day.

Evening Wrap-Up

*Not that I have already obtained all this, or have
already arrived at my goal, but I press on to take
hold of that for which Christ Jesus took hold of me.
Brothers and sisters, I do not consider myself
yet to have taken hold of it. But one thing I do:
Forgetting what is behind and straining toward
what is ahead, I press on toward the goal to win
the prize for which God has called me
heavenward in Christ Jesus.*
PHILIPPIANS 3:12–14

Setbacks are a part of life. Indeed, we all encounter
setbacks in all walks of life. But in his letter to the
Philippians, Paul reminds us to keep our eyes on
the prize. We are reminded to strain forward toward
the goal, and forget what lies behind. But all the
while, we can rest in the assurance that our lives
belong to Christ. And so we press on toward the
prize, striving toward wellness.

God of the Journey, *grant me patience with myself today
and each day when I deal with setbacks in my journey to
wellness. Remind me of Your constant presence in my life.*
In Your holy name, Amen.

Day 7:
Celebration!

Morning Reflection

Congratulations! We have completed one week on the journey toward managing hypertension! We have set goals, taken first steps, and made plans to deal with setbacks. Any journey is made more enjoyable and easier by celebrating our successes periodically. And so today, we should celebrate, and as we celebrate, we can look forward to the rest of the journey and the adventures of the weeks to come.

Faith Life
Today is a perfect day to celebrate the gift of your body. Go for a walk today and pay attention to the way that your legs move and the way that your breath moves in and out of your lungs.

Medical
Go for a walk today, and after ten minutes, check your pulse. Write down your heart rate and compare it to your resting heart rate.

Movement
Spend ten minutes doing some jumping jacks or another vigorous activity that might raise your heart rate. Try to make it an activity that you enjoy.

Work

As you sit at your desk at work, take a few minutes each hour to stand up. Do some squats or lunges to elevate your heart rate and strengthen your legs. This will give you a boost in energy and will give you some exercise during the day.

Emotional

On the journey to wellness, it is important to periodically reward yourself. But it is common for us to reward ourselves with food. Today, make a list of rewards for yourself that are not food related.

Family and Friends

Schedule a small celebration with your family and friends. Make a healthy meal at home, bringing your friends and families into the kitchen to share what you are learning on your journey.

Nutrition

Make a grocery list today that looks forward. Be sure to include lots of vegetables (fresh or frozen, or low-sodium canned), whole grains, and lean protein.

Evening Wrap-Up

*Sing to the L*ORD *a new song; sing to the L*ORD,
*all the earth. Sing to the L*ORD, *praise his name;*
proclaim his salvation day after day. Declare his
glory among the nations, his marvelous deeds
*among all peoples. For great is the L*ORD *and most*
worthy of praise; he is to be feared above all gods.
PSALM 96:1–4

At the end of this first week, we can remember that
God is walking this journey with us. Because God
walks the journey with us, God celebrates with us
as we celebrate our successes. On this journey to
wellness, God celebrates the strides that we make
toward wellness. Recall, moving forward from here,
that God made our bodies. God cares for our bodies,
and God cares when we care for our bodies. That is
reason enough to celebrate.

God of joy, help me to celebrate my successes today.
I know that You walk with me, and I know that You love me.
Give me the wisdom and peace of mind to celebrate.
In Your holy name, Amen.

Marcus's Story

Marcus was a healthy man when he joined Church Health Center Wellness. He had worked in the medical field most of his life, and after he retired, he took a job as a doorman at an apartment building to fight off boredom. While he enjoyed his doorman position, he missed getting regular exercise. He came to the Wellness Center and started an exercise routine that included lifting weights, riding the stationary bike, and walking and jogging on the treadmills.

Then, after several years of committed exercise, Marcus began to see more signs of his age. His blood pressure levels went up, and one day, he suddenly began experiencing pain in his shoulder. When he went to see his cardiologist, he was informed that he needed a quadruple bypass. Marcus was devastated that all his diligent exercise hadn't managed to protect his body from surgery. However, the surgery was a success, and Marcus made a fast recovery, returning back to work full-time before long.

Now, Marcus credits his speedy recovery to the many days and years he spent exercising at the Church Health Center. Although his bypass was a great shock to his system, he believes he wouldn't have been able to handle it if it hadn't been for his regular, steady exercise routine at Church Health Center Wellness. And now, he even volunteers his time to help others develop regular programs of exercise that they can commit to over the long haul.

Although his bypass was a great shock to his system, he believes he wouldn't have been able to handle it if it hadn't been for his regular, steady exercise routine at Church Health Center Wellness.

Day 8:
Habits

Morning Reflection

Hypertension is a disease that develops over time and is a product of both heredity (over which we have no control) and lifestyle (over which we can have control). But often, we think that our lifestyle is out of our control. This belief is partly because our day-to-day living is largely dictated by habits that are so deeply ingrained that we do not even realize what they are. Today, we will examine our habits.

Faith Life
Habits do not have to be bad. Today, make a list of your faith habits. For example, make note of praying before meals or reading the Bible in the morning.

Medical
This week we will focus on how you use your medication. Do you have a list of your medications? If not, make one today. Write or type a list of all of your medications and post it in an easy-to-find location, such as on the refrigerator.

Movement
Many of us do not move enough out of sheer habit. Today, go for a walk either after lunch or dinner to give your metabolism a little boost after your meal.

Work
What do you usually do when you get home after work? Do you watch television? Cook dinner? Today, take ten minutes or so to stretch before you start your usual "after-work" routine.

Emotional
Emotions are highly habitual. We can get into the habit of always feeling "busy" or "overwhelmed" or "stressed." Today, practice smiling twenty-five times. Just the act of smiling will trick your brain into feeling a different way.

Family and Friends
We have collective habits as well as individual habits. Today, think about the last time you were together with your family. Write about that time. Did you eat? Play games? Argue? What are your collective habits?

Nutrition
Most of us have formed rather poor nutritional habits, including drinking soda. Don't drink your calories today. Substitute water or unsweetened iced tea for sugary soda. (Hint: Even diet soda contains sodium, which can exacerbate hypertension.)

Evening Wrap-Up

Jesus left there and went along the Sea of Galilee.
Then he went up on a mountainside and sat down.
Great crowds came to him, bringing the lame,
the blind, the crippled, the mute and many others,
and laid them at his feet; and he healed them.
MATTHEW 15:29–30

Our habits are persistent and tough. It is difficult, even to the point of feeling impossible, to break or change these habits. But when we hang on to the right perspective, we can see that we have constant help from the God who walks with us. We are reminded that God cares for our bodies, and so God can help us care for them. After all, Jesus healed the lame, the maimed, the blind, and the mute. He healed their bodies, and He will help us heal our own bodies.

Healing God, help me to see the habits that are so deeply
ingrained in my life that I have become blind to them.
In Your holy name, Amen.

Day 9:
Triggers

Morning Reflection

Our habits do not work alone. Most of us have emotional and behavioral triggers that set into motion behaviors of which we may or may not be aware. As we identify those triggers, we can better control the behaviors that are contributing to an unhealthy lifestyle. Today, as we continue on the journey toward wellness, we will focus on ways to identify triggers and ways to deprive those triggers of their power over our behavior.

Faith Life
Quiet meditation, or "centering," is a wonderful tool to use in faith life. Today, sit for five minutes and concentrate on being quiet. Try to quiet your "inner voice" and content yourself with being still.

Medical
In the event of an emergency, someone should be able to find your medications. So, on the list of your medications that you made yesterday, make a note next to each name stating where it is stored (medicine cabinet, refrigerator, bedside table, etc.).

Movement
Today, each time you yawn during the day, do five jumping jacks. This will give you a boost of energy

when you are feeling tired and will give you a chance to try a new trigger.

Work
Today, try to identify your work triggers. For example, do you grab a cup of coffee or a soda every time you walk past the break room? Try keeping some herbal tea with you instead. This will help you stay hydrated and avoid becoming overcaffeinated.

Emotional
Emotional triggers are very strong and often difficult to detect. Today, take some time to write in your journal about what you do when you feel happy, bored, or sad. Knowing our reactions to these emotions can help us avoid unhealthy reactions when we have them.

Family and Friends
Family and friends provide us with some of our most pronounced triggers because families can easily fall into patterns of behavior that are largely out of our control. The next time you have a family gathering, try to focus on the fellowship and enjoyment rather than on food.

Nutrition
What do you reach for as soon as you feel a little bit hungry? Today, when you feel hungry, instead of snacking right away, wait until your hunger is at a "3" on a scale from 1 to 10 before you reach for a healthy snack.

Evening Wrap-Up

Come, all you who are thirsty, come to the waters;
and you who have no money, come, buy and eat!
Come, buy wine and milk without money and
without cost. Why spend money on what is not
bread, and your labor on what does not satisfy?
Listen, listen to me, and eat what is good,
and you will delight in the richest of fare.
Isaiah 55:1–2

When it comes to triggers, it can often feel like we are out of control. Behaviors and habits take over, and we end up eating when we had no intention of eating or sitting in front of the television when we had every intention of getting out for a walk. Why do you spend your money for that which is not bread? Isaiah is reminding us that God wants us to live lives full of nourishment.

Lord God, grant me strength today as I work to recognize
my triggers and change my habits. Help me to live a life
full of nourishment. In Your holy name, Amen.

Day 10:
Cleaning House

Morning Reflection

Our lives, generally speaking, are full of clutter. We are overwhelmed with schedules, tasks, and choices. Our pantries are overcrowded, often with food that is high in salt and sugar. As we continue on this journey, we need to clean house. Cleaning out our pantries, our bedrooms, and our offices can help to give us a clean slate, so to speak. Today, we will focus on clearing out the clutter to make room for lives that are healthy and wellness oriented.

Faith Life
Today, try again to sit, quietly meditating and centering yourself. Clear away the clutter of your mind and turn your focus to your breathing. Breathe in and let God in.

Medical
When was the last time you cleaned out your medicine cabinet? Lots of accidents can be avoided by disposing of expired and old medication. Today, take inventory of your medicine cabinet and throw out anything expired or unusable.

Movement
Take a half hour today and do some chores around the house. Vacuuming, mopping, dusting, and cleaning countertops can all get your heart rate up a bit. As an added bonus, when you're done, you will enjoy a clean house!

Work
Clear some space at work where you can store some healthy snacks, such as unsalted nuts or dried fruit. Then when you have a break, instead of going to the vending machine, reach for your healthy snacks and take a walk around the office.

Emotional
To calm some of the clutter in your mind today, set aside some time (even just ten minutes) to take a hot bath. As you soak, focus on breathing in and out, and let your body relax.

Family and Friends
Recruit some of your family and friends to clean your kitchen and especially your pantry today. Take the opportunity to throw out expired foods, as well as highly processed foods that are high in sodium, sugar, and fat.

Nutrition
Be careful of food products labeled "diet." Sometimes, these items have a significant amount of sodium. Your daily salt intake should be limited to no more than 1500 mg.

Evening Wrap-Up

It is written: "I believed; therefore I have spoken."
Since we have that same spirit of faith, we also
believe and therefore speak, because we know
that the one who raised the Lord Jesus from the
dead will also raise us with Jesus and present us
with you to himself. All this is for your benefit,
so that the grace that is reaching more and
more people may cause thanksgiving to
overflow to the glory of God.
2 Corinthians 4:13–15

As we clear the clutter from our pantries, our minds, and our desks, we make room for our own wellness. Paul, in his letter to the Corinthians, reminds us of the importance of spiritual renewal. When we get lost in the clutter of our lives, we cannot see even the possibility for renewal. So the first step is to make room for God.

Heavenly God, give me wisdom and patience as I make
room for You and for wellness in my life. In Your holy name,
Amen.

Day 11:
Attitude

Morning Reflection

When Marcus learned about his need for surgery, he was angry and frustrated. But afterward, he credited all those long hours of exercise with his ability to make a speedy recovery. When we find ourselves in the midst of a health crisis, it can be very easy to feel angry, frustrated, or tempted to give up. It may feel like there is nothing that we can do. This feeling, despite how strong it might be, is simply not true. But in order to truly change, we must have a positive attitude and acknowledge that change is possible, even though it may be difficult.

Faith Life
Take a short walk today. While you walk, pray that God will give you encouragement to continue on this journey. When you finish your walk, have a glass of water and remember that God has provided that water for you.

Medical
Remember that medications often have side effects—some are physical and some are emotional. If you are having emotional side effects (such as depression, anxiety, euphoria) or physical side effects, let your doctor know as soon as possible.

Movement
Exercise produces endorphins, which are "happy" hormones. Today, if you are feeling down or discouraged, do twenty-five jumping jacks or twenty-five lunges. The movement should give your mood a small boost.

Work
If you are having a difficult day at work, plan to do something you enjoy when the day is done (cook a delicious dinner, go for a walk outside, etc.). Write your plan on a note card that you can leave in a visible place.

Emotional
When you are tired and sleep deprived, having a positive attitude becomes even more difficult than it might normally be. Tonight, try to get to bed at a reasonable hour, allowing seven to eight hours for sleep.

Family and Friends
Your family and friends can be a wonderful source of encouragement when you are feeling discouraged. Today, make a list of five friends or family members who will help you at times when you need some encouragement.

Nutrition
Sometimes healthy eating is all about attitude. Think about a healthy food you didn't like as a child and that you like now. How did your attitude about that food change? What caused you to finally give that food a try?

Evening Wrap-Up

"Come to me, all you who are weary and burdened,
and I will give you rest. Take my yoke upon you
and learn from me, for I am gentle and humble
in heart, and you will find rest for your souls.
For my yoke is easy and my burden is light."
MATTHEW 11:28–30

Discouragement is a part of any journey, particularly when it comes to wellness. After all, most of us seek help and change only once we've been given a serious wake-up call. Because of that, it might seem easier to give up than to continue on the journey. But Jesus reminds us that He will lighten the burden. On this journey toward wellness, when we feel discouraged, we can turn to Jesus and hand over our burden. We can find all of the encouragement we need in God.

Ever-present God, grant me encouragement today.
As I continue on this journey, help me to hand over
my burdens to You. In Your holy name, Amen.

Day 12:
Wholeness

Morning Reflection

By this point in our journey, one thing should be clear: we are not focusing on only one aspect of wellness. This is because wellness is about the whole person— body and spirit. God created us as whole selves, and so as we continue on this journey, we ought to be turning our focus toward our whole self. Today, we will consider our whole selves as a part of God's creation, focusing on ways that we can appreciate and care for ourselves as a whole instead of individual, separate parts.

Faith Life
Take five minutes today to pray—but don't sit down! While you pray, wiggle your fingers and your toes. Take a deep breath in and let it out. Think about how your entire body can pray, rather than just your spirit.

Medical
In addition to prescription medication, do you take over-the-counter medication and/or vitamins? Be certain to include those on your list of medications for the refrigerator and the emergency contact.

Movement
Today, put on some music and spend some time dancing. Do not worry about looking silly. Feel your

body move—your head, your back, your legs. Have fun as you feel your body working as a whole unit together.

Work
Most of us work using one aspect of our personality more than other parts. Today, try to take five minutes at work and use another aspect of your body or personality. If you sit at a computer all day, go for a short walk. If you're on the phone, take a moment to stretch, and if you stand all day, find a quiet place to sit down.

Emotional
If you start feeling pulled in seventeen different directions today, pull yourself together by taking a hot shower. The water can drown out some of the noise of your life, and when you are finished, you will feel a little more "whole."

Family and Friends
Today, make a list of the different ways that your friends care for you. Has anyone ever brought you soup when you were sick? Do you have someone you can call when you are feeling down? Realize that your friends care for your whole self.

Nutrition
Remember that a truly balanced diet includes nutrients from a variety of sources. Today, make a meal including a variety of vegetables, grains, and proteins. Pay special attention to your sodium level!

Evening Wrap-Up

If the whole body were an eye, where would the
sense of hearing be? If the whole body were
an ear, where would the sense of smell be?
But in fact God has placed the parts in the body,
every one of them, just as he wanted them to be.
1 CORINTHIANS 12:17–18

Even though this journey is specifically about hypertension, this is truly a journey toward wellness, and we cannot get to our intended destination by ignoring our whole selves or favoring one part or another. In his letter to the Corinthians, Paul reminds us that God has arranged the members of the body to work in concert. God has created us whole. God has given us the gift of body and spirit—the gift of wholeness. So as we proceed on this journey, let us take care to remember our own wholeness.

God of healing, thank You for the gift of wholeness.
Help me today to continue on this journey as a whole
person, as You created me. In Your holy name, Amen.

Day 13:
Enjoyment

Morning Reflection

While the journey to wellness is not always smooth, we should find ways to enjoy ourselves. When we do this, we are more likely to keep a positive attitude and to stick with the journey. We are also less likely to become discouraged and to fall away from the journey if we are having a good time along the way. So today, we will turn our focus to finding ways to enjoy this journey to wellness.

Faith Life
While our faith life is important, it does not need to be devoid of enjoyment. Today, when you find yourself laughing or smiling, say a prayer of thanks.

Medical
Vitamins and supplements can help you manage symptoms and can help you avoid more potent medications (and their potential side effects). The next time you see your primary care provider, talk to him or her about supplements that you could take to improve your well-being.

Movement
Try not to look at exercise as a chore. Instead, try to find ways to move and be active that you enjoy. Go for a walk or play a game of basketball. Making

activities fun will increase your chances of staying active.

Work
While work is not often considered fun, finding aspects of your work that you enjoy can help. Today, make a list of some things that you enjoy about your work, even if it is as simple as liking the people you work with.

Emotional
If we do not spend time enjoying ourselves, we can easily become overwhelmed. Today, spend at least ten minutes doing something you truly enjoy. Try to take time each day to do something you like.

Family and Friends
Our family and friends can really help us to find enjoyment when we are feeling overwhelmed. Today, schedule an evening out with some friends and family. Go to a healthy restaurant and try something on the menu that you may not have had otherwise.

Nutrition
The next time you are invited to a party, take some baked tortilla chips and fresh salsa, or fresh-cut vegetables with hummus dip. This is a healthier alternative to potato chips and cream-based dip.

Evening Wrap-Up

Then Miriam the prophet, Aaron's sister, took a timbrel in her hand, and all the women followed her, with timbrels and dancing. Miriam sang to them: "Sing to the LORD, for he is highly exalted. Both horse and driver he has hurled into the sea."
EXODUS 15:20–21

After God liberated the Israelites from Egypt, we are told that both Moses and Miriam sang and danced. They praised God for all of the good that God had done. Though they were on the journey to the Promised Land, they still took the time to dance on the way. On our journey to wellness, we should also take the time to dance. Like Moses and Miriam, we can celebrate and enjoy our time on the journey. God does not wait to join us when we get to our destination. Rather, God is on the journey with us.

God of salvation, thank You for this journey.
Help me today and all days to enjoy the adventure.
In Your holy name, Amen.

Day 14:
Thanksgiving

Morning Reflection

Just as Miriam and Moses gave thanks in the wilderness when they had escaped Egypt, so should we give thanks each day on our own journey toward wellness. We have reached the end of the second week, and we are starting to get into the groove of this journey. When we stop and give thanks, we can gain a new perspective, realizing more fully what we've been given. So today, we give thanks for the past week and look forward to the weeks to come.

Faith Life
One of the most important aspects of our faith is thankfulness. Today, make a list of the things for which you are thankful. At the end of the day, say a prayer, reading the list.

Medical
Refilling prescription medications can be difficult to remember, but it is crucial for your health. If your pharmacy has an automatic refill program, use it. It will help you to fill your prescriptions on time.

Movement
When running errands, if you must stand in line, use the time to exercise your ankles and calves by doing

some calf raises. Rise onto your toes and let yourself back down. This will give you a little exercise and something to do while you stand in line.

Work
When you get frustrated at work, take a moment to breathe. Take a deep breath and say a short prayer of thanks. This can help you to take a step back and get some perspective before becoming overwhelmed.

Emotional
Gratefulness is an attitude that we can practice. When we remember what we have been given, some of the things that cause us stress might not feel quite so big. Today, when you start to feel stress, simply breathe and say the phrase, "I am grateful," before you move forward.

Family and Friends
Are you thankful for your friends and family? Do they know it? Today, take a moment and tell one (or more) of your friends and family members that you are thankful for their presence in your life.

Nutrition
Fruits and vegetables are healthiest when they are closest to their natural state. Today, eat two fruits or vegetables either raw or lightly steamed. Don't forget to give thanks before you eat!

Evening Wrap-Up

For I received from the Lord what I also passed on to you: The Lord Jesus, on the night he was betrayed, took bread, and when he had given thanks, he broke it and said, "This is my body, which is for you; do this in remembrance of me."
1 CORINTHIANS 11:23–24

At the end of this week, we are called to be thankful for the bodies God has given us and for the food that God provides. Paul reminds us that, even at the Last Supper, Jesus made sure to return thanks for the bread that He broke and shared with His disciples. So when we eat, we can be thankful that God breaks bread with us.

Giving God, make me thankful for all You have given me. In Your holy name, Amen.

Week 3

Arthur's Story

Arthur is a public school librarian who was described as kindhearted and gentle—but only by his wife! To other people, Arthur was stubborn, difficult, and even sometimes rude. After his wife became ill, Arthur became even more withdrawn and frustrating. He suffered from severe leg pain and hypertension and could barely walk. He also found that his wife could no longer prepare food for either of them and that he had to learn to cook to feed himself and his wife.

With no place else to go (and no other way of learning how to cook!), Arthur reluctantly signed up for the nutrition classes at Church Health Center Wellness. He began going every morning with the intent of learning the basics of how to cook but found himself enjoying the classes and taking better care of his health. The class instructor says that, though he started the class grumpy and complaining, his mood softened as he continued to attend.

When his wife died, the nutrition classes became a way to deal with his grief. His instructor suggested that he quit using salt, and so he filled his saltshaker with dried herbs and learned new recipes. Over some time, his blood pressure decreased. Recently, Arthur's nutrition classmates helped him plant an herb garden in his backyard. This past autumn, Arthur reaped his first harvest and hung his herbs to dry. He continues to learn new and better recipes and care for his hypertension using those fragrant herbs harvested from his garden.

The class instructor says that, though he started the class grumpy and complaining, his mood softened as he continued to attend.

Day 15:
Balance

Morning Reflection

Managing hypertension, as with all of wellness, is about finding balance. Balanced diet, balanced exercise, and life-work balances are all very important when it comes to living a wellness-oriented life. Of course, achieving balance is often easier said than done. Arthur wasn't able to find balance between his mood and his responsibilities at home until he found some friends at the Wellness Center. We all get busy and overwhelmed and then it is easy to fall back into old unhealthy habits and behaviors. This week, we will turn our focus to achieving and maintaining a balanced and wellness-oriented life.

Faith Life
Go for a walking meditation today. Walk for about ten minutes around your house, around your block, or even around your workplace. As you walk, make an effort to notice the wonderful way that your body is put together and the balance that helps you to walk.

Medical
Know your numbers. Talk to your doctor about what good blood pressure numbers are for you and what your goal is for a healthy reading. Write down your blood pressure number to remind yourself when you check your readings.

Movement
There is no movement without balance. Today, spend ten minutes balancing on one foot at a time. Balance as long as you can on one foot and then switch to the other. By balancing, you will build strength in your calves and ankles, as well as in your abdomen and back.

Work
Many of us talk about finding the right "balance" between work and personal life. Today, take five minutes and write about what the right balance looks like to you, whether you have currently achieved it or not.

Emotional
Balancing busyness with downtime is very important to maintaining emotional wellness. Today, take ten minutes to sit and relax. Take some deep breaths in and out. Close your eyes. Relax.

Family and Friends
All of us can lose our balance from time to time. It is at those times when it is most important to reach out for support. Today, go for a brisk walk with a friend or family member who might help to support you on your journey.

Nutrition
As with general wellness, good nutrition is mostly about balance and moderation. In particular, good nutrition includes appropriate portion size. Today,

keep a log of the things you eat and include the portion size. Remember that one portion of meat should be about the size of a deck of cards.

Evening Wrap-Up

*Instead, speaking the truth in love, we will grow
to become in every respect the mature body of
him who is the head, that is, Christ. From him the
whole body, joined and held together by every
supporting ligament, grows and builds itself up
in love, as each part does its work.*
EPHESIANS 4:15–16

Wellness means balance, particularly when it comes to managing hypertension. Hypertension comes about, in many cases, as a result of having an out-of-balance life. As we continue on the journey, we can try to find the right balance in life. In the passage from Ephesians, we are reminded of the balance with which God has created our bodies. Because of this balance, we can trust that God walks with us as we try to find that balance.

*God of Wisdom, thank You for the gift of this balanced body.
Walk with me as I try to achieve balance on this journey.
In Your holy name, Amen.*

Day 16:
Grace

Morning Reflection

How often do we cling to the idea that we must "do it all?" In an attempt to be strong, we sometimes refuse help and add stress to our lives when we might be better off accepting the helping hands offered to us. In particular, we sometimes forget that God is gracious and that God gives us grace, hope, and strength when we lean into that grace. Today, we will turn our focus to the grace that God offers us.

Faith Life
Today, read Matthew 19:26. Take five minutes and write about impossibility. Do any of your goals from Week 1 feel impossible? How might God give you the grace to face even seemingly impossible tasks?

Medical
Many communities have clinics that can help people who can't afford medical care. Today find a community center or clinic that can offer you a helping hand with your needs or someone you know.

Movement
Today, spend ten minutes stretching. Try to touch your toes, reach your arms across your chest, and stretch your back. If your muscles are cold, do not stretch too far!

Work
Is your office break room always full of treats such as birthday cake, donuts, or bagels? Offer a balance to some of these unhealthy snacks by bringing healthy snacks to share, such as a fruit and vegetable plate.

Emotional
Learning to manage stress is very important to managing hypertension. Today, take a slow walk, focusing on your breathing and letting go of the things that leave you overwhelmed.

Family and Friends
Do you and your family have dinner together? Today, plan a family dinner made up of mostly vegetables. Include a lean protein and a small serving of whole grains (such as brown rice, barley, or whole-wheat pasta).

Nutrition
Depriving yourself entirely of the foods you love makes you more likely to binge. Balance a strict food intake and calorie counting with an occasional small treat. Today, treat yourself to a sensible treat, such as a small serving of dark chocolate or a scoop of low-fat frozen yogurt.

Evening Wrap-Up

My heart is not proud, Lᴏʀᴅ, my eyes are not haughty; I do not concern myself with great matters or things too wonderful for me. But I have calmed and quieted myself, I am like a weaned child with its mother; like a weaned child I am content. Israel, put your hope in the Lᴏʀᴅ both now and forevermore.

Psᴀʟᴍ 131:1–3

Managing hypertension requires achieving an overall balance between medications, lifestyle, diet, exercise, stress, and other factors. All of this can be overwhelming and can even cause us more stress than the stress we began with! But if we can remember to quiet ourselves, God offers us hope and balance, even when we have difficulty finding that balance ourselves. On some days, our job is to simply quiet our souls and give in to the grace that God offers.

Gracious God, grant me the grace and quiet to find balance on my journey to wellness. In Your holy name, Amen.

Day 17:
Balanced Senses

Morning Reflection

Our perspective of wellness is often limited to numbers on a scale. But wellness is about much more than weight. Wellness is about incorporating all the senses. God, after all, has given us the blessing of sight, smell, sound, taste, and touch. It makes sense, since God has created us with all of those senses, that a wellness-oriented lifestyle would include all of our senses. Today, we will turn our focus to the senses with which we have been blessed.

<u>Faith Life</u>
Remember that God shows up in every aspect of our lives, including our food. Today, before each meal, say a prayer. Thank God for the flavors and the colors in your food.

<u>Medical</u>
Remember that your current medical state is closely related to your family history. Today, write out a brief medical history of your family. Pay special attention to hypertension and heart disease. Keep your medical history close by, along with your list of medications.

<u>Movement</u>
Go for a walk today, and as you walk, observe all of

the colors, smells, and even tastes. Pay attention to the air on your skin and the movement of your body. Say a prayer of thanks for all of those sensations as you move.

Work

If you become bored at work today, try not to resort to eating. Instead, take a moment and make a list of fifteen things that you can see, smell, feel, hear, or taste. Then say a small prayer of thanks.

Emotional

When our emotions flare up and we become overwhelmed by stress, our blood pressure goes up. In managing hypertension, we must try to limit that surge of blood pressure. Today, practice deep breathing to bring down your blood pressure during times of stress.

Family and Friends

Healthy relationships can bring balance to your life in many ways but especially by offering fellowship and fun. Today, call a friend or a family member and have some fun by dancing to music or shopping at a farmers' market for good local fresh produce.

Nutrition

In managing hypertension, it is important to limit salt intake. Today, try adding flavor to your food by adding herbs and spices, such as basil, parsley, or rosemary. Add flavor to a sandwich by adding watercress or cabbage instead of lettuce.

Evening Wrap-Up

*When John, who was in prison, heard about the
deeds of the Messiah, he sent his disciples to ask
him, "Are you the one who is to come, or should
we expect someone else?" Jesus replied,
"Go back and report to John what you hear
and see: The blind receive sight, the lame walk,
those who have leprosy are cleansed, the deaf
hear, the dead are raised, and the good news
is proclaimed to the poor."*
MATTHEW 11:2–5

God created us with all of our senses. And then,
Jesus saw fit to grant hearing to the deaf and sight
to the blind. God has filled this world with beauty
and has blessed us with the senses to be able to
appreciate that beauty. When we live wellness-
oriented lives, we live lives that are well balanced
in all of God's creation.

*God of Creation, You have filled my life with
beautiful colors, tastes, and smells.
Help me to live my life in the fullness of Your creation.
In Your holy name, Amen.*

Day 18:
Our Comfort Zone

Morning Reflection

As we work to change our lives, we often find ourselves thrust out of our comfort zone and into foreign territory. Arthur never would have joined a cooking class, but he had to learn to enjoy and utilize this new opportunity. On this journey to wellness, we are asked to try new foods, to move in new ways, and to push limits that have been confining. But wellness is about changing an entire lifestyle, which includes venturing out beyond our limits. Today, we will focus on moving beyond our comfort zones and striking balance in the wellness zone.

Faith Life
Read Exodus 3, where God appears to Moses in the burning bush. When you have finished, spend five minutes writing about being called out of your comfort zone. Do you feel God's assurance, "I will be with you"?

Medical
It is important for you to know the symptoms of a stroke: weakness in one arm or leg, loss of feeling on one side, blindness in one eye, difficulty talking, loss of balance. If you have any of these symptoms—or know of someone who is experiencing them—you should seek medical help immediately.

Movement
A healthy exercise regimen consists of building our aerobic strength, muscular strength and endurance, and flexibility. Today, do three sets of ten wall push-ups to start building your upper-body strength.

Work
When you begin to feel tired or bored at work, pay attention to your posture. Good posture helps you to breathe, increases strength in your back and abdomen, and can give you a boost of energy when you need it.

Emotional
Leaving your comfort zone can cause a great deal of anxiety or even panic. Today, if you begin to feel anxious about leaving your comfort zone, slow down, take several deep breaths, and tell yourself out loud that you are safe.

Family and Friends
When we are making changes in our lives, we might find ourselves in opportunities to make new friends. Today, say hello to someone you rarely talk to, or try to think of a person with whom you could develop a new friendship.

Nutrition
Eating a wellness-oriented diet means leaving behind food habits that may be comfortable and even comforting. Today, try a new food, paying particular attention to the salt content. (Hint: Do not add any salt until after you have tasted a dish.)

Evening Wrap-Up

*But now, this is what the L*ORD* says—he who
created you, Jacob, he who formed you, Israel:
"Do not fear, for I have redeemed you; I have
summoned you by name; you are mine.
When you pass through the waters, I will be
with you; and when you pass through the
rivers, they will not sweep over you.
When you walk through the fire, you will not
be burned; the flames will not set you ablaze."*
ISAIAH 43:1–2

As we continue on this journey toward wellness,
we are asked time and again to try new things. We
ask our bodies to move with exercise. We ask our
taste buds to appreciate different flavors. We are
asked to step out of our comfort zone in any number
of ways, each of which might be frightening. But
Isaiah assures us that God is with us.

*Faithful God, walk with me today as I move into unfamiliar
places. Help me to step outside of my comfort zone.
In Your holy name, Amen.*

Day 19:
Purpose

Morning Reflection

As we progress on this journey, we need to step back and reevaluate our progress, looking particularly to the initial goals that we set in the first week of this journey. In other words, we must reconnect with our purpose for being on the journey. Keep in mind that purposes will differ from person to person and may even change for one person from day to day or moment to moment. Today, we will touch base once again with our purpose for the journey.

Faith Life
What were your goals for your faith life in Week 1? Today, reread your goals, and then spend five minutes writing about your progress. Have any of your goals changed? Have you made progress where you hadn't expected?

Medical
Hypertensive people are at a higher risk for heart attack. The symptoms of a heart attack include: chest discomfort; discomfort in one or both arms, back, neck, or jaw; shortness of breath; cold sweats; light-headedness; and nausea. If you experience any of these symptoms—or know of someone who is experiencing them—seek medical attention immediately!

Movement
In Week 1, you went for a walk. Go for a walk today. Do not exhaust yourself, but push yourself to walk as far as you can. Write in your journal the progress that you have made.

Work
Today, take a copy of your list of medications, vitamins, over-the-counter medications, and family history to keep at work. Keep the list in an accessible place.

Emotional
Connecting with our purpose on the journey can help us to gain stability and perspective as we go through periods of change. Today, spend ten minutes writing in your journal about your purpose on this wellness journey.

Family and Friends
Family and friends can be strong reminders of the purpose that we set for ourselves. Today, have a healthy meal with your family or some friends, and enjoy the social anchor that you have in your support system.

Nutrition
What has changed in your diet since you started on this journey? Take a moment and write out your grocery list from this week. Compare it with the grocery list you made during Week 1. What has changed? What has stayed the same?

Evening Wrap-Up

*There is a time for everything, and a season
for every activity under the heavens: a time to
be born and a time to die, a time to plant and a
time to uproot, a time to kill and a time to heal,
a time to tear down and a time to build, a time to
weep and a time to laugh, a time to mourn and
a time to dance, a time to scatter stones and a
time to gather them, a time to embrace and
a time to refrain from embracing.*
ECCLESIASTES 3:1–5

As we pause and consider our purpose at this
particular moment on this particular journey, we
must remember that our purpose fits into God's
creation quite beautifully, as we are reminded in
this passage from Ecclesiastes. God gives us life
and purpose, which fit beautifully with God's larger
creation. It is that purpose that can anchor us when
we feel discouraged or lost on the journey.

*Loving God, help me to remember purpose—both mine
and Yours—on this journey. In Your holy name, Amen.*

Day 20:
Change

Morning Reflection

This journey is all about change. Change, even the most strived-for change, comes with its fair share of challenges. Arthur's life was changed dramatically with the death of his wife and his new friendships at the Church Health Center. With all of the changes that are happening now all at the same time, we can get thrown a little off-kilter. So today we will turn our focus on how to keep our balance in the midst of this change.

Faith Life
Do you have a "go-to" Bible verse that you return to when you need comfort or support? Today, spend ten minutes reflecting on one verse that anchors you. Remember that you have anchors even in the midst of change.

Medical
If possible, have a place at work where you can keep medication that you need during the day, instead of taking your medication with you to work each day. Make sure they are well labeled!

Movement
Today, if you are running errands, park your car in the parking space farthest away from the entrance

to the store. Add steps to your day by forcing yourself to walk farther to the store.

Work
When work becomes topsy-turvy, it can be very easy to stress-eat without even recognizing what you are doing. Today, if you start to feel overwhelmed at work, don't head for the vending machines; head for the door! Take a short break outside, breathe in some fresh air, and let your body relax before getting back to work.

Emotional
Many of us, in the past, have dealt with the discomfort of change by eating. Today, make a list of things that you can do to give yourself comfort that will help on your journey. Go for a walk, for example, or read a book.

Family and Friends
When was the last time you contacted an old friend? Write your friends a note, e-mail, text message, or just call them up on the phone.

Nutrition
Salads are definitely healthy, but be careful of the dressing and cheese! Use low-fat cheese, and substitute cream-based or mayonnaise-based dressings (like ranch or Thousand Island) with a vinaigrette or even just some vinegar and oil with a little pepper and oregano.

Evening Wrap-Up

Remember your leaders, who spoke the word of God to you. Consider the outcome of their way of life and imitate their faith. Jesus Christ is the same yesterday and today and forever. Do not be carried away by all kinds of strange teachings. It is good for our hearts to be strengthened by grace, not by eating ceremonial foods, which is of no benefit to those who do so. . . . Through Jesus, therefore, let us continually offer to God a sacrifice of praise— the fruit of lips that openly profess his name.
HEBREWS 13:7–9, 15

Change happens in life. But when we are actively working to change multiple aspects of our lives, change can actually take us by surprise and knock us off balance. In the letter to the Hebrews, we are reminded that all things change—except for Jesus Christ. "Jesus Christ is the same yesterday and today and forever." When we feel we have lost our anchor in a sea of change, Jesus Christ is the anchor.

Life-sustaining Lord, thank You for Your constancy and Your unchanging love and support. Today in the midst of change, remind me that You are my anchor. In Your holy name, Amen.

Day 21:
The Halfway Point

Morning Reflection

Congratulations! At the end of this week, we are now midway through this six-week journey. At the halfway point, we may feel both excitement and discouragement: encouragement for the distance we have covered, and perhaps some discouragement for the distance yet to travel. Because of that discouragement, we need to stock up on encouragement so that we do not run out of steam. We're in the middle of the race, and now is the time to dig deep and tap those extra stores of endurance to continue on the journey.

Faith Life
Endurance comes with peace, and peace often comes with quiet. Today, practice sitting quietly. Take time to sit quietly and breathe. Reflect on the journey to this point and how God has been present with you.

Medical
What are your long-term health goals? Keep in mind that quick fixes in medicine are generally not long-term solutions. The next time you have a doctor's appointment, talk to your care provider about your long-term health goals.

Movement
Today, do some jumping jacks. Try a set of fifteen, take a one-minute break, and then do it again. Try that three times throughout the day. Remember that in order to build endurance, we must occasionally push limits.

Work
When you take your break at work, do you crave a specific food? This may be habitual eating. Today, if you feel hungry at work, drink some water or snack on some chopped, fresh vegetables instead of heading for the vending machines.

Emotional
Marathon runners will tell you that endurance is at least as emotional as it is physical. Today spend five minutes concentrating on breathing and repeat to yourself that you can continue on this journey. Try not to tell yourself that this is something that you cannot do.

Family and Friends
Friends are an important part of encouragement. Today, schedule a dinner with some of your friends who will give you encouragement for the journey.

Nutrition
For dessert tonight, instead of a sugar-rich and fatty dessert, try grilling some fruit kabobs and eating them with low-fat yogurt or ricotta cheese. Grilling the fruit will bring some of the natural sugars to the surface and will add a little natural sweetness.

Evening Wrap-Up

And pray in the Spirit on all occasions with all kinds of prayers and requests. With this in mind, be alert and always keep on praying for all the Lord's people. Pray also for me, that whenever I speak, words may be given me so that I will fearlessly make known the mystery of the gospel, for which I am an ambassador in chains. Pray that I may declare it fearlessly, as I should.
EPHESIANS 6:18–20

The journey to wellness and to managing hypertension is a lifelong one. This six-week journey is halfway done, but as far as we have come, we still have an equal distance to go. At this point in the journey, it can be easy and unsettling to look at how far we have yet to travel. In his letter to the Ephesians, Paul gives us encouragement to pray at all times. That prayer gives us strength for the journey.

Lord God, thank You for bringing me this far on the journey. Give me strength and endurance to continue. In Your holy name, Amen.

Alejandra's Story

The first time Alejandra came to the Church Health Center, she parked in the space reserved for the handicapped drivers and walked in with a cane. She struggled with arthritis and chronic pain, and her care provider recommended that she lose weight because her blood pressure had reached a dangerously high point.

At first Alejandra was only able to exercise in the therapeutic pool, which is designed specifically for people who have difficulty with movement and walking. She struggled to get to and from the Wellness Center but tried to make it to at least one class every other day. After several months of exercise with the support of the warm water, she was able to begin walking on the treadmill, riding the stationary bike, and doing strength training. She still enjoys the relaxing workout of the pool classes but has been able to lose more weight in other exercise classes.

Now, Alejandra parks wherever she wants! She can walk most of the time without any assistance, and her arthritis and hypertension have improved dramatically. Though she continues to meet with her doctor every four months, Alejandra is proud to say that her blood pressure is back in the safe range, and she is maintaining her health.

Now, Alejandra parks wherever she wants!

Day 22:
God's Creation

Morning Reflection

Alejandra relied on water, a part of God's creation, to help her exercise. We so often look to wellness as simply an individual journey to health, but on this journey, we should consider that wellness is about being good stewards of God's creation. After all, we are created in God's image! Caring for our own bodies, more than vanity or even health, is about caring for God's creation. Today and this week, we will focus on how we can care for ourselves as a part of all of creation.

Faith Life
Psalm 34:8 reads, "Taste and see that the LORD is good; blessed is the one who takes refuge in him." Take five minutes and write about finding God in many aspects of creation, including your food.

Medical
Good medicine is preventive medicine. Write the names of your medicines and dosages on 3" x 5" index cards and put them in your wallet or purse. This way you will always have them on hand.

Movement
Exercising in a pool can be a great way to shake up your exercise routine. Today, take a dip in a pool or

investigate where you might find an accessible pool at a gym or community center.

Work
Are you able to see outside from your place of work? Today, bring some inspiring pictures to work to give you a break from the indoors when you need it.

Emotional
The sound of water can be calming to our emotions. Today, take a few moments to listen to the sound of running water or the waves of the ocean and think about how this can have a calming influence on your emotions.

Family and Friends
Today, go to a park with your family and friends. Enjoy being outside in God's creation with them. Instead of focusing on food, focus on the fun and beauty of creation.

Nutrition
For managing hypertension, whole grains are particularly important. In fact, even one serving of whole grains a day can help prevent the exacerbation of hypertension. Today, replace white bread, refined cereals, or pasta with whole grains: brown rice, whole-grain cereals, or whole-wheat bread, crackers, and pasta.

Evening Wrap-Up

*In the beginning, Lord, you laid the foundations
of the earth, and the heavens are the work
of your hands. They will perish, but you remain;
they will all wear out like a garment. You will roll
them up like a robe; like a garment they will be
changed. But you remain the same, and your
years will never end.*
HEBREWS 1:10–12

God's creation is precious not only to God but to each of us. As we continue on this journey, we can be encouraged and inspired by God's beautiful creation. But as eternal and as beautiful as God's creation seems to be, God is even more so! God is constant and powerful. And as we progress, we can find comfort and solace in God's eternal presence with us, for God never ends.

*Powerful God, thank You for the wonder of Your creation.
Help me today to appreciate Your creation, including
my own body, and to care for it the best I can.
In Your holy name, Amen.*

Day 23:
The Sun

Morning Reflection

As we prepare for the day, what do we do? For most of us, our morning looks something like this: shower, shave, get dressed, pack a bag, jump in the car, and drive to work. Once we get to work, we often spend our time inside, before heading back home to watch a television show, make dinner, or do laundry. We rarely take the time during the day to bask in the light of God's creation: the sun. Today we will celebrate the sun as it gives energy to our lives.

Faith Life
If you get stuck in traffic today, rather than cursing the people around you, try praying. Today, pray, "God, thank You for the gift of light."

Medical
Do you smoke? If so, it is time to stop. Smoking makes hypertension worse and puts you at a higher risk for stroke, heart attack, heart failure, and even kidney failure. Talk to your care provider about ways that you can get help for smoking cessation.

Movement
Spend some time outside today, walking or even going for a light jog. Even if it is cold outside, put on some layers and get outdoors.

Work
Enjoying the sun can be particularly difficult at our jobs, but our work is not just at our job. Today, do some work outside. Wash your car, mow your lawn, work in your garden. You'll get some sun and some exercise!

Emotional
The sun can provide a much-needed emotional lift, as well as vitamin D. Today, find ten minutes to sit outside in the sun and practice deep breathing. Feel the sun's warmth and try to let your body relax as you sit.

Family and Friends
Go for a walk outside with a friend or family member. Try to enjoy the outdoors and the company of someone who cares for you.

Nutrition
If you have not done so yet, write down your sodium intake for one or two days this week. How close are you to 1500 mg?

Evening Wrap-Up

*And God said, "Let there be light," and there was
light. God saw that the light was good, and he
separated the light from the darkness. God called
the light "day," and the darkness he called "night."
And there was evening, and there was
morning—the first day.*
GENESIS 1:3–5

God created the sun, giving us a great gift. However,
too often we are so busy we forget to step into the
light at all! Instead, we should be enjoying the
wonders of God's creation. The truly amazing thing
is if we do enjoy God's creation responsibly, we will
also be healthier. Enjoying the sunshine responsibly
will help lower our stress and encourage us to
exercise. Furthermore, the sun simply feels good.
What a wonderful gift!

*Light in the darkness, help me today to make the most of
Your creation. Especially help me to enjoy the light that
You have given me. In Your holy name, Amen.*

Day 24:
The Air

Morning Reflection

There has been a great deal of talk about air pollution, and it is true that pollution is a problem. But air is also a gift—one that we often forget about. God has given us the gift of air to breathe. Air is *breath*, air is *smell*, air is a *breeze* on a hot day, and air is *warmth* coming from the fire on a cold day. So today, we are going to celebrate the wellness that comes with the air.

Faith Life
There are dozens of verses in the Bible about how God uses the wind. Today, read John 3:8, and when you encounter the wind today, take it as a reminder of God's Spirit moving in the world.

Medical
Make taking your daily medicine easy to remember. Use weekly pill boxes so you only have to refill it once a week. Keep this in an easy-to-remember location.

Movement
Today, try to walk someplace where you would normally drive. Get some great exercise by walking and keep just a little of those pollutants from getting into the air.

Work

If you feel anxiety at work, try to do some deep breathing. Take just a minute and focus on controlling your breathing. It will help to lessen your anxiety and will give you a boost of energy and focus.

Emotional

Air is a very important part of stress relief. Today, spend five minutes sitting with your back straight, breathing. Breathe in through your nose and out through your mouth. If you start to feel light-headed, try to relax your chest and stomach muscles.

Family and Friends

Prepare a meal today with your family or some friends and enjoy all of the aromas that you produce in the kitchen. The smells of food all come from the gift of air.

Nutrition

In addition to increased vegetables, three servings of low- or non-fat dairy products daily have been shown to lower blood pressure. Today, try eating a cup of non-fat yogurt or cottage cheese for a snack and drink a glass of skim or 1 percent milk with lunch.

Evening Wrap-Up

*And God said, "Let there be a vault between
the waters to separate water from water."
So God made the vault and separated the water
under the vault from the water above it. And it
was so. God called the vault "sky." And there was
evening, and there was morning—the second day.*
GENESIS 1:6–8

Air is breath and is truly that which gives us life.
But it often goes unnoticed. We cannot see air, but
we can feel it in a breeze on a hot day or in heat on
a cold day. We can smell it coming from a delicious
meal. So today is a perfect day to stop and take
notice of God's wonder in the creation of the air.

Spirit-filled God, *thank You for giving me breath.
Help me today to slow down and notice the gift and the
beauty of the very air that I breathe.* In Your name, Amen.

Day 25:
Water

Morning Reflection

We already saw how helpful water was for Alejandra. Water covers about 70 percent of the earth's surface, and our own bodies are made up of 57 percent water on average. Water also provides us opportunities to have fun—while swimming or on vacations to lakes and beaches. Rain gives us not only the possibility for growing food but also the lush and beautiful trees and flowers in our neighborhoods. And yet, most medical experts agree that we generally do not drink enough water. Today, we will focus on God's gift of water.

Faith Life
The next time it rains, try to think of the rain as a blessing. Today, write a prayer thanking God for the blessing of water.

Medical
Obesity tends to reduce the percentage of water in your body, which contributes to hypertension. Today, count the glasses of water (or clear, unsweetened, non-caffeinated fluid) that you drink. You should be drinking about eight 8-ounce glasses a day.

Movement
Swimming is excellent exercise. It is gentle on your

joints and works just about every muscle group in your body. Today, if you have access to a pool, go for a swim—even spending ten minutes in the water will give you some great exercise.

Work
Instead of drinking soda during breaks, try drinking water. The sugar and caffeine in soda can actually leave you dehydrated and feeling lethargic. Water will replenish your bodily fluids and will leave you with more and lasting energy, instead of just a sugar rush.

Emotional
Most of us shower in the morning. Today, to relax, take a five-minute shower at the end of the day. The noise from the shower will help to drown out the noise of the day, and the heat from the water will help to relax your muscles.

Family and Friends
Serving water with meals is a great way to meet your daily water goals (at least eight 8-ounce glasses). Today, when you have dinner with your family, put a pitcher of water on the table with the rest of the meal.

Nutrition
If you want a beverage other than water, drink some unsweetened herbal tea or fruit juice, but stick with 100 percent fruit juice. (Keep in mind that fruit juice—even 100 percent fruit juice—has fairly high sugar content.)

Evening Wrap-Up

And God said, "Let the water under the sky be gathered to one place, and let dry ground appear." And it was so. God called the dry ground "land," and the gathered waters he called "seas." And God saw that it was good. Then God said, "Let the land produce vegetation: seed-bearing plants and trees on the land that bear fruit with seed in it, according to their various kinds." And it was so.
GENESIS 1:9–11

Water is one of the most significant and powerful parts of God's creation. It is one part of God's creation that all of life on earth needs in order to survive. Water has the power of life. But we also know that water has the power of destruction. We know the story of Noah and the great flood. So as we move on from this day, we can appreciate the power and the beauty of this aspect of God's creation.

God of nourishment, help me to remember that water is an important part of my journey to wellness. Give me the eyes to see You in water. In Your holy name, Amen.

Day 26:
Our Bodies

Morning Reflection

This week, we have been reflecting on particular aspects of God's creation. So often we think of God's creation as that which is outside ourselves—trees, water, air, sun. Though that is true, we also sometimes forget that we ourselves are integral to God's creation. Today, we remember that God created us along with the rest of creation. So caring for God's world includes caring for ourselves—which, of course, is what this journey is all about.

Faith Life
Today, as you pray, wiggle your toes and say a prayer of thanksgiving for your toes. Then bend your knees and thank God for your knees. Continue moving and praying until you get all the way up to your hair.

Medical
If you have any kind of recurring pain in your shoulder, make sure that you mention that to your care provider. Shoulder pain can be a hidden sign of heart disease, and if you have hypertension, your risk of heart disease is fairly high.

Movement

At this point on your journey, you should be getting aerobic exercise for thirty minutes most days of the week. Today, remember to stretch before and after you exercise to avoid injury.

Work

Work often requires repeating the same motion monotonously. When you take a break, spend five minutes doing something completely different from what you usually do. For example, if you sit at a computer typing most of the day, stand up and do jumping jacks.

Emotional

How do you feel about your body? Many of us are not happy with the way we look. Spend five minutes today writing about what you like about your body. Remember, your body is created by God!

Family and Friends

Many of our self-esteem issues come from directing hatred toward our own bodies. Today, ask a friend or family member to tell you what they like about your body.

Nutrition

Today, instead of eating red meat (like beef) with your meal, try a lower-cholesterol, leaner option, such as turkey, chicken, or fish. (Hint: Do not eat the skin!)

Evening Wrap-Up

He said to them, "Why are you troubled, and why
do doubts rise in your minds? Look at my hands
and my feet. It is I myself! Touch me and see;
a ghost does not have flesh and bones,
as you see I have." When he had said this,
he showed them his hands and feet.
LUKE 24:38–40

Our bodies are an important part of God's creation.
Any time we are tempted to dismiss the body as
insignificant, we should come back to this passage
in Luke. God became human in a body, and Jesus
died a bodily death and rose again. He ate, He drank,
He touched, and He was touched. All of those truths
are significant to the way that we interact with and
care for God's creation.

God of my life, thank You for this body that You have given
me. Please help me to remember what a gift my body is.
In Your holy name, Amen.

Day 27:
Community

Morning Reflection

When we think of God's creation, we often think of that first chapter in the book of Genesis: light, water, sky, land, plants, animals, and finally humans. We do not often think of community as a part of God's creation. But community has been a part of God's world since Adam and Eve. We are surrounded by community, and we live in community. So today we will focus on how we can care for, and be cared for by, community.

Faith Life
Are you a part of a faith community, such as a church or a prayer group? Do you think you are the only person struggling with hypertension? Today, spend five minutes writing about ways that you can get your faith community on a journey to wellness.

Medical
Hypertension can cause problems with your eyesight. If you have frequent headaches or vision problems, such as sudden vision loss (even if it is regained quickly), tell your care provider, and schedule a routine eye exam.

Movement
Housework burns calories and helps you feel like you've accomplished something. Today, take on a task in your home that you don't usually do. For example, take out the trash, dust your bookshelves, clean the bathroom or the kitchen. Then, invite someone over to enjoy your efforts!

Work
Your coworkers are a community, whether you want them to be or not. Today, try bringing in a healthy treat for your office—a fruit plate or some fresh vegetables.

Emotional
Do you ever feel lonely? Being part of a community is very important to our overall wellness. Today, spend ten minutes writing about your community. Remember that communities come in many forms— families, book clubs, churches, etc.

Family and Friends
Have a meal with your closest community—your family or close friends. Try to focus on enjoying the fellowship more than the food.

Nutrition
Do not be a member of the "Clean Plate Club." Today, pay attention to your feelings of hunger as you eat. Let your hunger, rather than your plate, dictate how much you eat.

Evening Wrap-Up

*Every day they continued to meet together in the
temple courts. They broke bread in their homes
and ate together with glad and sincere hearts,
praising God and enjoying the favor of all the
people. And the Lord added to their number
daily those who were being saved.*
ACTS 2:46–47

We are not created to exist alone. From the very
beginning, we have been created to live with each
other in community. After all, God created Adam
and Eve to keep each other company. Community
offers us companionship, support, encouragement,
and courage when we need it. And at the center of
those communities is God, whose love is a gift to
each of us individually and in community.

*God of relationship, help me to appreciate the communities
that You have created around me. Give me the wisdom
to see the blessing of community in wellness.
In Your holy name, Amen.*

Day 28:
Our Spirit

Morning Reflection

Congratulations. We've made it to the end of the fourth week! We are two-thirds of the way along the journey. At this point, we are finding ways to improve our wellness. We should be starting to notice changes in our body and spirit. Today we will think about how change in our body can also change our attitude, our emotions, and our spirit.

Faith Life
What do you think a healthy spirit is? Today, take ten minutes to pray and then write a few sentences about what *healthy spirit* means to you.

Medical
Kidney disease is a possible side effect of prolonged hypertension. Fortunately, it is mostly reversible with lifestyle change and medication. If you notice constant swelling, particularly in your lower legs, more frequent urination (particularly at night), or if you have difficulty urinating, be certain to mention this to your care provider.

Movement
Helping a neighbor do yard work or even to move is a wonderful act of kindness and generosity, and it can get your heart rate up and burn calories! Today,

try to help a friend, family member, or neighbor with a project.

Work
If you find yourself standing in one place for a period of time (making copies, talking on the phone, waiting for lunch to heat up), spend that time doing squats or calf raises.

Emotional
We often expect perfection of ourselves. The trouble with such expectations is that we are simply not perfect, and we can become demoralized. Today, write for ten minutes about a time when you have expected perfection from yourself.

Family and Friends
Today, recruit some family members and friends to help you with a project that you have been putting off—rearranging furniture, painting a room, mowing the lawn. Getting things accomplished is a great way to bond and lift spirits generally.

Nutrition
Avoid frying vegetables or cooking them in cream sauces. Try using a healthier preparation, such as grilling, baking, or steaming. This will help maintain maximum flavor without adding extra fat, salt, and cholesterol.

Evening Wrap-Up

But the fruit of the Spirit is love, joy, peace, forbearance, kindness, goodness, faithfulness, gentleness and self-control. Against such things there is no law. Those who belong to Christ Jesus have crucified the flesh with its passions and desires. Since we live by the Spirit, let us keep in step with the Spirit.
GALATIANS 5:22–25

Today, we have reached the end of this fourth week, and we should be noticing some changes in our day-to-day lives. We are becoming more active, adopting a healthier diet, and hopefully appreciating many aspects of God's creation. With all of these changes happening, it is inevitable that we will find our spirits changing along with everything else. And as Paul writes in his letter to the Galatians, the change in spirit can come from God's Spirit.

Sustaining Spirit, help me to see You at work in me as I continue on this journey to wellness. In Your holy name, Amen.

Week 5

Dora's Story

Dora came to the Church Health Center Medical Clinic a few years ago. She had diabetes and hypertension, a fairly standard combination of ailments, but Dora herself was no ordinary patient. A deeply spiritual woman, Dora asked if she could give her doctor a blessing at the end of their appointment. "I like to know that my doctor has the Lord looking out for him," she said. The doctor, having never been blessed by a patient, agreed. Dora shot out of her chair and grabbed his head with both her hands, praying words of strength and wisdom for him.

From that day forward, Dora was one of the most committed patients of the Church Health Center. She arrived early for every appointment, began exercising at the Wellness Center, and continued to see her doctor—blessing him each and every chance she got. She brought the power of healing into the Church Health Center as she sought treatment for her physical ailments and healing for her spiritual ills.

Her efforts in exercise and nutrition extended her husband's life for many years.

Dora brought the power of healing into the Church Health Center as she sought treatment for her physical ailments and healing for her spiritual ills.

Day 29:
Variety

Morning Reflection

This journey is full of change and variety that we may not even expect. Each one of us experiences the journey in a different way, and one person may even experience the journey differently from day to day. The variety, while it can be a challenge, is really a blessing. We can learn from variety, and in variety, we can sometimes see God and ourselves in a new light. So today we will look at variety as a blessing and as a necessary part of the journey.

<u>Faith Life</u>
We have all experienced variety and change in our faith life. Take ten minutes today and write about a time in your faith journey when you started heading one direction, but life or God pointed you down an unexpected path.

<u>Medical</u>
Are you on medication? Have you been feeling better? Do not stop taking any medication until you have discussed it with your primary care provider. Stopping medication suddenly can lead to relapse, drug resistance, or unexpected side effects.

Movement
A wonderful way to get some exercise and appreciate God's creation is to go for a hike. Find a park in your area that has some trails available for this purpose. Don't forget to bring water and a healthy snack.

Work
At work during your lunch break, find some stairs and climb up and down them several times. This gives you a great aerobic workout without even needing to go to the gym.

Emotional
We are approaching the end of this six-week journey. Do you have different expectations now than you did when you started? Spend five minutes today writing about your current expectations for the journey.

Family and Friends
Family and friends can be our constants when other things in life are unpredictable. Today, make a healthy meal for your family or some friends. Enjoy the food, but focus on the company and conversation.

Nutrition
For managing hypertension, it is generally recommended that you consume no more than six ounces of meat a day. Today, try to go the entire day without adding meat. Try some vegetarian recipes using beans, nuts, or soy for protein.

Evening Wrap-Up

*The law of the Lord is perfect, refreshing the soul.
The statutes of the Lord are trustworthy,
making wise the simple. The precepts of the Lord
are right, giving joy to the heart. The commands
of the Lord are radiant, giving light to the eyes.
The fear of the Lord is pure, enduring forever.
The decrees of the Lord are firm, and all of them
are righteous. They are more precious than gold,
than much pure gold; they are sweeter than honey,
than honey from the honeycomb.*
Psalm 19:7–10

In many ways, we have reached the summit of this
journey, and we are heading back down the other
side of the mountain. As we continue, we have the
gift both of looking back on what we have learned
and looking forward to the progress we have left.
At this point, we can enjoy the variety that God
provides as a part of the journey. As the psalmist
writes, God revives the soul.

*Loving God, thank You for such a varied and beautiful
creation. Help me to appreciate Your variety as I continue
on the journey. In Your holy name, Amen.*

Day 30:
God in Our Midst

Morning Reflection

The process of making lifestyle changes for any reason can be overwhelming. In our case, making lifestyle changes to manage hypertension can be particularly overwhelming. We can experience a great deal of pressure, both from within and from without, to make the changes stick, or to look better, or to feel better every day. If we don't feel 100 percent every day of the journey, we can feel guilty or even feel like quitting. Today we will explore the ways that God walks with us on this journey.

Faith Life
Take ten minutes today and reflect on and write about the darkest moment in your faith life. Did God find you there? How?

Medical
While it is sometimes important to lose weight in order to manage your hypertension, it is also possible to lose weight too quickly, resulting in malnutrition or loss of muscle and bone mass. Talk with your doctor about setting healthy and reasonable weight-loss goals.

Movement
This week, try stepping up your aerobic exercise by doing ten jumping jacks before you go out for a walk and when you get back. This will help get your heart rate up so you start out your walk with a higher heart rate.

Work
Instead of going out to eat or getting lunch out of a vending machine, bring in a lunch made from your leftovers from last night's dinner. It is almost guaranteed to be healthier, and it is much less expensive!

Emotional
Have you had any setbacks recently? Today, take five minutes to write about your setbacks, and then let them go. Move forward from here.

Family and Friends
Soon, these six weeks will be done, and it will be time to find your own rhythms and patterns. Today, write down the names of a few friends or family members who might be willing continue with you on the journey to wellness.

Nutrition
Some fats are necessary for balanced nutrition. Healthy fats can be found in avocado, seeds and nuts, olive oil, and fish. Today, prepare a meal using mostly healthy fats (no fried food or butter).

Evening Wrap-Up

The virgin will conceive and give birth to a son,
and they will call him Immanuel
(which means "God with us").
MATTHEW 1:23

We continue on this journey, through both setbacks and successes, and we are reminded today that God walks with us. Remember that Jesus is called Emmanuel—God with us. Because Jesus is human, God has walked on this earth. God can now walk with us as we walk this journey. This is why we call our God *incarnate*. God became human so that God could be with us on all of our journeys.

Ever-present God, thank You for the gift of Your Son, Jesus.
Help me to honor His body and mine on this journey.
Continue to walk with me, I pray.
In Your holy name, Amen.

Day 31:
The Seasons

Morning Reflection

Our journey to wellness is a lifelong journey. On the journey, we will pass through many seasons. As Ecclesiastes reminds us, to everything there is a season. That is a part of the journey. But as the seasons change, so do we. Sometimes we mourn the season past, and sometimes we are excited about the season to come. Sometimes we feel a little bit of both. Whatever our reaction, though, the changing of seasons happens. Today, we will turn our focus to the coming and going of seasons.

<u>Faith Life</u>
We can see God in all of the seasons, wherever and whenever we are. But sometimes it is easier than other times. In which season can you see God most easily? Take five minutes and write a prayer for that season.

<u>Medical</u>
Knowing your BMI, or body mass index, can help you as you make changes to improve your hypertension. Today, find some information about calculating your BMI, and try to learn what your number is.

Movement

Different seasons allow different kinds of exercise. During the summer, you can go swimming; in the autumn, you can play in the leaves; in winter, you can shovel snow. Today, try to engage in a season-specific activity.

Work

Most workplaces have periods that are busy and periods that are slower. Whatever your work environment is like at this moment, find five minutes to breathe and stretch a little.

Emotional

Are your expectations that your lifestyle changes will be all-or-nothing? Today, take five minutes to write in your journal, reminding yourself that setbacks and individual "failures" are just seasons. If we persevere, they will pass.

Family and Friends

Are there seasons (such as the holiday seasons) when you spend more time with your family? Take a few minutes today and brainstorm some ways to make your family gatherings healthier, knowing what you know now about wellness.

Nutrition

A wonderful way to add variety to your diet is to buy seasonal fruits and vegetables. They will be fresher than out-of-season produce and will also cost less.

Evening Wrap-Up

He makes springs pour water into the ravines;
it flows between the mountains. They give
water to all the beasts of the field; the wild don-
keys quench their thirst. . . . He makes grass grow
for the cattle, and plants for people to cultivate—
bringing forth food from the earth: wine that glad-
dens human hearts, oil to make their faces shine,
and bread that sustains their hearts. . . . He made
the moon to mark the seasons, and the sun
knows when to go down.
Psalm 104:10–11, 14–15, 19

God has built times and seasons into creation. The psalmist reminds us of just how beautiful the design of God's creation is. "He made the moon to mark the seasons." God has designed creation such that the seasons are simply part of the rhythm of creation. And as we are a part of God's creation, we, too, have seasons. Even as we walk on this journey toward wellness, we experience seasons of change.

Lord God, thank You for the beautiful seasons
You've granted Your creation. Give me the wisdom and
flexibility to adjust to the seasons with grace.
In Your holy name, Amen.

Day 32:
Sounds

Morning Reflection

Though this journey is particularly a journey toward hypertension management, our focus is on the whole self. After all, hypertension is an illness that results from multiple factors—heredity, lifestyle, diet. And so on this journey, we have taken into account many factors to strive toward wellness. Today, we will turn toward another aspect of our lives—sound.

Faith Life
What is your favorite sound in the world? Today write for five minutes about that sound. What does the sound remind you of? Where does God fit into that sound?

Medical
There are many different types of blood pressure medication. Today, if you are taking medications, make sure you know the types of medications you are on, not just their names. If you have questions, call your doctor and ask.

Movement

Sound can be such an important part of movement, but we often ignore it. Today, as you go for your walk, listen to some music. Try to follow the rhythm as you go.

Work

If it is appropriate, put on some soft music while you work, using either small speakers or headphones. Listening to music can help to pass time and can also lift your mood or relax you.

Emotional

Sound can help you identify and deal with your moods. Today, take five minutes and write down ten sounds that you find comforting and calming. Then, the next time you feel overwhelmed or stressed, imagine one of those sounds to calm yourself down.

Family and Friends

When you gather family and friends for a holiday or special occasion, think about playing games instead of focusing entirely on food. That way the gathering is more about being in each other's company rather than eating.

Nutrition

Beware of frozen dinners. Quick though they may be, they are often loaded with sodium. Sometimes the diet versions are a little better, but there is no guarantee. Be sure to read the labels before consuming.

Evening Wrap-Up

*Shout for joy to God, all the earth! Sing the glory
of his name; make his praise glorious. Say to God,
"How awesome are your deeds! . . . All the earth
bows down to you; they sing praise to you, they
sing the praises of your name."*
PSALM 66:1–4

Sound can be a reminder of God's grace and presence in our lives. Noises can also be ways that we praise and worship God. The psalmist writes, "Make a joyful noise." Can there be a more joyful noise than a healthy person moving and enjoying the movement? What would happen if we considered the sound of our feet on the pavement on the same level as praise and worship songs? Perhaps we would walk a little more! As we move forward, let us remember that God loves us and wants us to be healthy.

*Dear God, thank You for the gift of sound. Help me to hear
the music all around me, even in my own footsteps.
In Your holy name, Amen.*

Day 33:
Sight

Morning Reflection

As we continue on this journey, our experience of the old things may begin to change. For example, our old eating habits may become less appealing as we get used to eating healthier meals. Riding the elevator may seem a missed opportunity to climb the stairs. Parking a car may look like an opportunity to get in a bit of a walk before grocery shopping. Our perspective changes as our priorities change, and it can be like being granted sight after being blind.

Faith Life
Do you have potluck dinners at your church? The next time you have a potluck dinner, take a healthy dish instead of a more typical dish. (For example, bring a fresh fruit salad instead of a pie.)

Medical
Today, take a few minutes to critique your vision, and if necessary, make an appointment to have your eyes checked or your prescription updated. Also keep in mind that hypertension can cause vision problems, and let your ophthalmologist know about your hypertension.

Movement
Go for a walk today. Walk for as long as you can manage and take in the sights of the world around you. Try to notice the difference in your walking now from when you started.

Work
If you feel rushed before the workday even begins, take five minutes to pray or visualize the day ahead. This will help relax you and keep you centered.

Emotional
Do you have any visual cues that are connected to your emotional state? For example, what do you feel when you look out the window and see snow? Or the sight of a fire in the fireplace? Today, take five minutes and write about some of the most emotionally powerful images in your life.

Family and Friends
Today, for fun, get out some old pictures of you and your family. Try to remember when the pictures were taken. Let the pictures inspire storytelling and camaraderie around a healthy meal.

Nutrition
Many vegetable juices tout five servings of vegetables in a single cup, but buyer, beware! Those juices might contain up to 653 mg of sodium (about half of what your daily intake should be). Instead of vegetable juice, simply nibble on a small bag of baby carrots and sliced cucumbers.

Evening Wrap-Up

"While I am in the world, I am the light of the world." After saying this, he spit on the ground, made some mud with the saliva, and put it on the man's eyes. "Go," he told him, "wash in the Pool of Siloam" (this word means "Sent"). So the man went and washed, and came home seeing. His neighbors and those who had formerly seen him begging asked, "Isn't this the same man who used to sit and beg?"
JOHN 9:5–8

The Bible is full of stories of the blind regaining their sight. On this journey, however, we are not trying to restore our eyesight; we are learning how to see again. On this journey, we are learning to see wellness as the goal. We are learning to see our world differently, from our friends to our food.

God of sight, with Your help my perspective can change. Give me the vision of wellness. In Your holy name, Amen.

Day 34:
The Fruits of Wellness

Morning Reflection

As we approach the last week of our journey, we may begin asking ourselves what we have gotten from the journey. But what we miss when we ask that question is that the journey to wellness is a continual journey. In continuing to strive toward wellness, the more the fruits of wellness manifest themselves. When we live wellness-oriented lives, we are better able to participate in the fullness of life.

Faith Life
Today, look back on your journey. Meditate for a few minutes, remembering where you started on the journey. Where have you found God on this journey?

Medical
If you forget to take your medication for one dose, do not take a double dose. Instead, call your primary care provider and ask whether you should take a dose immediately or wait until it is time for the next dose to get back on track.

Movement
Today, step up your aerobic exercise by carrying small weights with you on your walk. If you do not

have weights, fill a couple of bottles with water and carry those with you on your walk.

Work
How has this journey impacted your work life thus far? Have you noticed changes in your attitude, your work ethic, your productivity? Consider how you have changed your work life today and take note of your improvements.

Emotional
Today, keep a list of the different emotions that you feel throughout the day. If you notice a lot of "stressful" feelings, do some meditating or take a bath at the end of the day.

Family and Friends
What do celebrations with your family and friends look like? Lots of sugary, fatty foods? Today, write out a plan for your next celebration. Include healthy foods and drinks.

Nutrition
Instead of buying canned soups, try making a big pot of soup, either stove-top or in a slow cooker. Freeze the portions that you do not eat right away. This way, you can control the amount of sodium that goes in, and you can flavor the soup to your taste.

Evening Wrap-Up

Praise be to the God and Father of our Lord Jesus Christ! In his great mercy he has given us new birth into a living hope through the resurrection of Jesus Christ from the dead, and into an inheritance that can never perish, spoil or fade. This inheritance is kept in heaven for you, who through faith are shielded by God's power until the coming of the salvation that is ready to be revealed in the last time. In all this you greatly rejoice, though now for a little while you may have had to suffer grief in all kinds of trials.
1 PETER 1:3–6

In most Christian communities, we are fond of talking about a new birth. Usually a new birth refers to a spiritual death and rebirth in Christ. But this journey to wellness also gives us a new birth, in that it offers us new life. Wellness affords us the opportunity to live a new life, and God walks into that new life with us.

Living God, give me the wisdom today to embrace a new life on this journey. In Your holy name, Amen.

Day 35:
Healing

Morning Reflection

Today we reach the final day of the fifth week. We are coming to the end of our six-week journey, but the larger journey is really just beginning. Think of Jesus' forty-day walk in the wilderness. It was not His entire life, but the preparation for the rest of His life. Our six-week journey is the preparation for the wellness journey after the six weeks are completed. The journey to wellness is a journey toward healing. Today, we will focus on how wellness heals.

Faith Life
Have you ever been healed? Keep in mind that healing can happen in many forms. Today, write about what you think it means to be healed.

Medical
Did you know that some over-the-counter medications contain sodium? Because managing hypertension requires following a low-sodium diet, be sure to read the ingredients on everything you consume, including medication. Look for ingredients such as sodium carbonate or bicarbonate.

Movement

Exercise is incredibly healing. Today, spend ten minutes warming up your muscles with some jumping jacks or jogging in place. Then spend at least five minutes stretching your muscles.

Work

Do you ever go out for lunch as a part of your work? When you do, make sure to order a lower-sodium option, such as fish or a salad without cheese.

Emotional

Physical healing means very little without emotional healing. Take ten minutes and write about a time in your life when you experienced emotional healing, such as a time when you have forgiven or been forgiven.

Family and Friends

A large part of any healing is our support system. Today, have a conversation with the members of your family and friends who are an important part of your support system. Tell them what healing on this journey looks like for you.

Nutrition

Cheese is the number-one source of saturated fat in the American diet. It is also fairly high in sodium and cholesterol. Instead of adding cheese to your dishes today, try adding flavor with some lemon zest or a little vinegar.

Evening Wrap-Up

*Praise the LORD. How good it is to sing praises to
our God, how pleasant and fitting to praise him!
The LORD builds up Jerusalem; he gathers the
exiles of Israel. He heals the brokenhearted
and binds up their wounds. He determines the
number of the stars and calls them each by name.
Great is our Lord and mighty in power;
his understanding has no limit.*
PSALM 147:1–5

Many of us begin a journey toward wellness when we
are sick, tired, and frustrated. We come to the journey
searching for healing, and we experience small
changes that lead slowly to healing. As we change
our lives, we can rest in the assurance that God walks
with us and God does heal us, even as we work to
change our lives.

*Healing Lord, thank You for walking this journey with me.
Help my body to heal as I continue on my journey
toward wellness. In Your holy name, Amen.*

Week 6

Eloise's Story

In the late 1980s, Eloise was paralyzed after an injury. She was left unable to work and was having difficulty caring for herself. She came to the Church Health Center a few years later with hypertension and depression. As with most people who come into the Church Health Center, Eloise was given a diet and exercise regimen and was monitored by the staff on each visit.

Though she still gets around in a wheelchair, Eloise's hypertension is under control, she has lost weight and gained muscle mass in her arms. Even better, she is no longer in the grips of the crushing depression that brought her to the Church Health Center twenty years ago.

What made the difference? In Eloise's case, it was the fact that she surrounded herself with people who cared about her and supported her. One of her care providers wrote about her, "I have found Eloise to be very independent, and I suspect her life is better more because of her own strengths than anything we did. Still, her story is a great example of what the Church and people of faith are capable of doing for each other. She is an example that broken bodies do not have to keep broken spirits from healing."

What made the difference? In Eloise's case, it was the fact that she surrounded herself with people who cared about her and supported her.

Day 36:
Our Conversion Stories

Morning Reflection

We all have conversion stories of some sort, where we came to a new or different understanding of our faith. Some conversions are instantaneous, and others are longer stories, similar to the filling of a bucket drop by drop. However it happens, those experiences can be turning points in our lives. They exist in all aspects of our lives, even though we tend to most closely associate conversions with our faith life. When it comes to our journey toward wellness, there are many small conversions—small changes—that amount to a turning point.

Faith Life
Today, spend five minutes writing about your conversion story. Was it gradual or sudden? What do you feel changed in your life?

Medical
At this point in the journey, you may want to increase your exercise level. If you are going to engage in any kind of a rigorous exercise program, make sure that you talk to your doctor first. He or she can help you safely exercise.

Movement

By now, it would be a good idea to step up your exercise routine. Go for a slightly longer walk, using weights, and do jumping jacks when you return. Do not forget to drink water and stretch!

Work

At work today, during a break, grab a couple of coworkers and take a walk. Walk around your office, around the block, or go to a mall and walk for a while. Just give yourself a little activity and company to break up your day.

Emotional

Many times, quick conversions are what we could call mountaintop experiences. But the real work is done in the valleys. Today, write about times when you have been on the mountaintop and how those experiences translate to the work in the valleys.

Family and Friends

Sometimes conversions can feel very lonely. Today, go out and have fun with some friends or family members. They will help to remind you that you are not alone.

Nutrition

Canned vegetables and fruits can be easy and fast alternatives to fresh produce. However, they often come packaged in a good deal of salt and/or sugar. If you are trying to make a quick dish, try using frozen vegetables rather than canned. They usually have less sodium and preservatives.

Evening Wrap-Up

As he neared Damascus on his journey,
suddenly a light from heaven flashed around him.
He fell to the ground and heard a voice say to him,
"Saul, Saul, why do you persecute me?" "Who are
you, Lord?" Saul asked. "I am Jesus, whom you are
persecuting," he replied. "Now get up and go into
the city, and you will be told what you must do."
ACTS 9:3–6

Most of us are very familiar with Saul's conversation story. He got knocked off his horse, blinded, and came out the other side a different man—with a different name. While Paul's story is very dramatic, it is important to realize that his conversion was only the beginning of his ministry. In a similar way, this six-week series is really only the beginning of the wellness journey. That God walks with us.

Lord God, help me today to embrace my conversions,
however they come to me. In Your holy name, Amen.

Day 37:
Knowing Ourselves

Morning Reflection

As we are growing into new people on this journey, we must take some time to become reacquainted with ourselves. As we change our habits and our tastes, we can begin to see the person in the mirror as somewhat of an unfamiliar person. As we move toward wellness, we need to take a step back from the journey to become acquainted with the people we have become and are becoming. Today, we will turn our focus to knowing ourselves.

Faith Life

What does it mean to love yourself? Spend five minutes writing about loving yourself. Keep in mind that God loves you and has commanded you to love your neighbor as yourself, meaning you must love both your neighbor and yourself.

Medical

If you choose to drink alcohol, talk to your care provider about the amount of alcohol you can safely consume. Most medical experts recommend no more than two alcoholic beverages a day for men and no more than one for women. Remember that alcohol consumption contributes to hypertension.

Movement
Today, as you cook dinner or wait for a phone call, etc., do three sets of ten wall push-ups. Try to lower yourself a little deeper with each push-up. You should feel your heart rate increase a bit and feel the muscles in your arms and abdominals working.

Work
If you must go out for lunch at work, try to avoid eating fast food. Instead, try to find a place where you can order lean protein and vegetables that are not fried.

Emotional
At the end of the day today, find some time to care for yourself. Take a bath, read a book, call some friends to hang out. Relieving stress and caring for yourself is a crucial element to managing hypertension.

Family and Friends
When you plan activities with your family and friends, try going to a park, playground, or museum instead of going immediately to a restaurant. This way you will have some kind of physical activity built into your outing. Many cities have "free days" at museums for a low-cost activity.

Nutrition
Sodium, saturated fat, and cholesterol can be hidden in foods that otherwise look healthy. Do not count on pictures or names for nutrition information. Remember, read before you buy!

Evening Wrap-Up

You have searched me, LORD, and you know me.
You know when I sit and when I rise; you perceive
my thoughts from afar. You discern my going out
and my lying down; you are familiar with all my
ways. . . . For you created my inmost being; you
knit me together in my mother's womb. I praise
you because I am fearfully and wonderfully made;
your works are wonderful, I know that full well.
PSALM 139:1–3, 13–14

No matter how much change we go through in our lives, God is constant, and we are fully known to God. God has "formed our inward parts." Whatever changes we make in our own lives, and whatever setbacks and successes we experience, God continues to know us, and God continues to travel this journey with us.

Creator God, I know that I am fearfully and wonderfully
made. Help me to see You in myself.
In Your holy name, Amen.

Day 38:
The Next Steps

Morning Reflection

As we approach the end of this six-week journey, it is important for us to look into the future and set up our next steps. When we began this journey, we set up "first steps," considering our goals and trying to find ways to meet those goals in these six weeks. Now that the six weeks are nearly over, it is time to set new goals and make new plans for the next phase of the journey.

Faith Life
Today, take five minutes and reflect on how far you've come in this journey. Then turn your focus to the future.

Medical
Earlier in this journey, we taught you how to take your heart rate. Take it again today and see how you have improved in these few weeks.

Movement
Try to begin incorporating movement into your daily mundane activities. For example, if you run to the store to buy a gallon of milk, carry the milk with you instead of putting it in a cart. Then, while you stand in line, do some alternating bicep curls with it.

Work
Bring an insulated lunch bag to work with some raw prepared vegetables such as celery, carrots, and red bell peppers to snack on when you get hungry. If you want to add a little spice, throw in a few radishes as well.

Emotional
Moving forward from here may be intimidating. Today, make a list of stress-relieving activities that you have learned over the past six weeks.

Family and Friends
Your family and friends will be very important to your journey. Today, try to set up a regular walking time with (at least) one of your friends or family members. Having a regular time will help you get in (and stay in) the habit of walking.

Nutrition
Aim for five servings of vegetables in a day. To get all of those servings, try serving at least two different vegetables with dinner. Tonight try a cooked option (like steamed broccoli) and a raw option (such as some sliced red peppers or a salad).

Evening Wrap-Up

Therefore, I urge you, brothers and sisters,
in view of God's mercy, to offer your bodies as a
living sacrifice, holy and pleasing to God—this is
your true and proper worship. . . . Just as each of
us has one body with many members, and these
members do not all have the same function,
so in Christ we, though many, form one body,
and each member belongs to all the others.
ROMANS 12:1, 4–5

The journey toward wellness is truly about transformation and hope. As we continue to change our habits to embrace wellness, we are being continually transformed. That transformation will bring us a greater appreciation for our bodies and for the masterful way that God has put us all together. And our relationship with God will be transformed as well.

Merciful God, help me today as I begin to look down the road. Grant me hope and encouragement for what is to come. In Your holy name, Amen.

Day 39:
Fellow Travelers

Morning Reflection

We are in the final days of our six-week program. As we approach the finish line, we must take some time to consider life after this part of our journey has come to a close. In particular, today we will be focusing on the people in our lives who touch us on the journey. Our faith communities, doctors, friends, and families are all integral parts of the journey, even if they do not walk the exact path we do.

Faith Life
Does your faith community have Sunday school programs? Today, consider starting up a Sunday school program that is centered on the wellness journey. Encourage other members of your faith community to live wellness-oriented lives.

Medical
Remember that medication is not a magical pill. When your physician writes a prescription for a medication, ask questions about what lifestyle changes you should be making along with the medication to be healthier.

Movement

Today, before your family sits down for dinner, go for a walk together. Doing some exercise before you eat will make you feel better and will give you a better gauge on your appetite.

Work

If there is someone at your work who shares your particular lunchtime, and perhaps is interested in eating healthy meals, adopt that person as a lunch buddy. Take turns bringing in new, healthy dishes to try.

Emotional

When we feel alone, we can become despondent, and it can really halt our progress on the wellness journey. Today, spend five minutes writing about the many ways in which you are not alone.

Family and Friends

Your family and friends can be of great support, but it can also be good to seek support from people who are going through similar experiences. Support groups exist at gyms and wellness centers as well as online. Find a group that you can join.

Nutrition

No matter how much you want to lose weight, do not start a fad diet. While they may help you lose weight, fad diets generally do not promote overall wellness or lifelong change, as they often include unbalanced meal plans.

Evening Wrap-Up

*My command is this: Love each other as I have
loved you. . . . You did not choose me, but I chose
you and appointed you so that you might go
and bear fruit—fruit that will last—and so that
whatever you ask in my name the Father will give
you. This is my command: Love each other.*
JOHN 15:12, 16–17

We have already said on this journey that we were
created to live in community. We are not made to
walk alone. Jesus sets for us a perfect example of
living in community and loving our fellow travelers.
As we continue on the journey from here, remember
to continually reach out to your fellow travelers.
People who are on similar paths can offer tremendous
love and support to one another.

*Living Lord, thank You for those I have met on my journey.
Thank You for the support and the love shown to me.
In Your holy name, Amen.*

Day 40:
Forty Days!

Morning Reflection

Today is Day 40—congratulations! You have made it forty days! Over the past six weeks you have gained the skills necessary to continue on your journey toward hypertension management. Setbacks will probably happen from time to time, but in the last six weeks, you have set a foundation that you can return to when needed. The journey to hypertension management may take you to unexpected places, but wherever wellness takes you, it is sure to lead to a fuller and more abundant life.

Faith Life
At the end of this six-week journey, we can begin to imagine life beyond this series. In particular, we can think about abundant living, which, after all, has been the goal. Take five minutes today and write about what you think abundant living means to your life now.

Medical
If you change health care providers, try to get to know them while you are healthy. It is much easier for doctors to treat you when they know what "healthy you" is like.

Movement
In celebration of reaching the fortieth day of managing hypertension, put on some music and dance around your house. Laugh as you want to and let go of your inhibitions for a while.

Work
If you need to go out to lunch for work, ask for a "to go" box to come out with your food. If the portions are larger than what is healthy (as is the case at most restaurants), put half of your order in the box before you eat.

Emotional
Today, try to rest. When we are tired, overworked, and sleep deprived, our body responds to stressors, causing us to hang on to weight and contributing to hypertension.

Family and Friends
Today, prepare a meal for your friends and family that you have never prepared before. Get your guests to help you prepare the meal, chopping vegetables or stirring the pot as things cook.

Nutrition
When you go out to eat, ask for meals to be prepared with no salt. That way, you can control the salt that goes onto a dish, and you will know your sodium intake for that meal.

Evening Wrap-Up

*Arise, shine, for your light has come, and the glory
of the LORD rises upon you. See, darkness covers
the earth and thick darkness is over the peoples,
but the LORD rises upon you and his glory appears
over you. Nations will come to your light, and
kings to the brightness of your dawn. Lift up your
eyes and look about you. . . . Then you will look
and be radiant, your heart will throb and swell
with joy; the wealth on the seas will be brought to
you, to you the riches of the nations will come.*
ISAIAH 60:1–5

Our lives are full and rich and abundantly blessed.
The journey to wellness is simply about living up to
the abundant grace that God has already granted
us. We can thrill and rejoice in God because God has
granted us beautiful bodies and abundant life. Recall
that Jesus promises us life, and life in abundance.
Through this journey to wellness, we can take Him
up on that offer.

*Sustaining God, help me today to see and take advantage
of the abundant life that You have given me.
In Your holy name, Amen.*

Day 41:
Review

Morning Reflection

Now that the forty days are over, today will be a day of review. When we started out this journey, we had to assess where we were in order to set goals for the journey. In a similar manner, we have to assess where we are again, so that we can know where we need to go from here. We need to see our successes as well as our setbacks, so that we know that on which we still need to work.

Faith Life
When we started, you wrote ten words describing your faith life. Again, take five minutes and write ten words describing your faith life now. Then compare the two lists. What has changed? What has stayed the same?

Medical
Has your medical situation changed? Take a few minutes today and look at how far you have come in the last six weeks.

Movement
Go for a walk today and walk as far as you can walk. How far could you walk the first time you did this? Can you feel the improvement in the way your body is reacting to the walking?

Work
Prevent office burnout by taking little breaks when you can, Just five or ten minutes away from your desk will help you feel refreshed.

Emotional
What has changed in your emotional wellness? Take a look at your emotional highs and lows from Week 2. Do you still have similar highs and lows, or has your overall emotional pattern changed a bit?

Family and Friends
What have your family and friends thought about your journey? Can they see a difference in you? Take a moment today and ask one or two of them for feedback.

Nutrition
In the first week, you made a list of the foods that you like to eat. Can you expand that list any after six weeks? In particular, can you include more healthy meals on that list?

Evening Wrap-Up

*I have fought the good fight, I have finished
the race, I have kept the faith.*
2 Timothy 4:7

The last six weeks have been challenging in a variety of ways. You have been asked to try new things, from food to exercises. You have been asked to step outside your comfort zone and explore emotions that most of us do not take the time to explore regularly. But the journey—at least this part of the journey— is finished. And you have finished this race. For that, you ought to be very proud and thankful. You have run the race, and God has been running right beside you. Remember as you continue from this point, God runs the race with you. God gives us all strength and endurance when we most need it, and God cheers when we cross the finish line.

*God of my life, thank You for the gift of wellness.
Help me to continue on this journey with endurance
and bravery. In Your holy name, Amen.*

Day 42:
Looking Ahead

Morning Reflection

With the six weeks completed, it can certainly feel as if the journey is over. However, as has been said before, the journey has really only just begun. The journey to wellness is never over. Life will offer us many surprises along the way, and it will be part of the journey to adapt as life happens. Today as we close this chapter on the journey, we look ahead to continue the lessons learned.

Faith Life
As you continue on this journey, remember to take time to pray or meditate each day. Prayer and meditation can keep you connected to your purpose and your anchor.

Medical
Take all medication exactly as prescribed, and do not be afraid to talk to your doctor about anything. The best way to stay medically healthy is to have open communication with your physician.

Movement
Move everywhere. Find ways to add a few steps to your day in everything that you do. A great goal would be to add 200 steps to each day, which will help your body to burn calories more efficiently.

Work

Try to find time in your days to exercise—even a little bit. It will help break up the monotony of the day and will help you to add a few steps. Also, avoid office junk food. Instead, opt for healthy snacks and lunches.

Emotional

Find and remember ways that you can relieve stress. Take a hot bath, go for a walk, read a book. Just find something that works for you and do it every day. The more you relieve your stress, the better you will feel, and the healthier you will become.

Family and Friends

Remember that your family and friends are your support system. When you are struggling, do not be afraid to lean on them for support, and when you have succeeded, do not be afraid to celebrate with them.

Nutrition

Make your calories count. Enjoy all of the wonderful colors and flavors of God's creation as you prepare meals using whole grains, a variety of fruits and vegetables, and lean meats—but let yourself splurge on occasion!

Evening Wrap-Up

*Finally, brothers and sisters, whatever is true,
whatever is noble, whatever is right, whatever
is pure, whatever is lovely, whatever is
admirable—if anything is excellent or
praiseworthy—think about such things.
Whatever you have learned or received or heard
from me, or seen in me—put it into practice.
And the God of peace will be with you.*
PHILIPPIANS 4:8–9

It has been a long journey to this point, but you have been given many tools to continue on your way. You will find other tools to add to your toolbox, and you will have setbacks. But remember that God walks with you, and God can grant you peace, even when you have a difficult time finding it for yourself.

Lord of the future, be with me as I continue on this journey. Help me to remember the things I have learned and help me to continue learning. I will continue to strive to honor my body and my whole self, Your creation. In Your holy name, Amen.

Recommended Reading and Resources

Websites

The Church Health Reader, www.chreader.org. Here, you can find interviews with leaders and thinkers; tips and advice on running effective ministries; faithful reflections on living with disease; reviews of relevant resources; recipes for larger groups such as soup kitchens and church suppers; and tested curricula such as our own Walk & Talk. Our mission is simple: to make you and your church healthier in body and spirit. It begins with each of us making healthier decisions for ourselves and our churches. The Church Health Reader is here to help you do just that.

American Heart Association, http://www.heart.org/HEARTORG/. The mission of the American Heart Association is to "build healthier lives free of cardiovascular disease and stroke."

National Institute of Health, http://www.nih.gov/.

National Heart, Lung, and Blood Institute, http://www.nhlbi.nih.gov/.

Books

Regaining the Power of Youth at Any Age, by Kenneth H. Cooper. This book features a scientifically based program that will guide you to a higher level of physical and mental fitness that you may have believed impossible to attain.

What to Eat, by Marion Nestle. Nestle walks readers through every supermarket section—produce, meat, fish, dairy, packaged foods, bottled waters, and more—decoding labels and clarifying nutritional and other claims (in supermarket-speak, for example, "fresh" means most likely to spoil first, not recently picked or prepared), and in so doing explores issues like the effects of food production on our environment, the way pricing works, and additives and their effect on nutrition.

The Inner Game of Stress: Outsmart Life's Challenges and Fulfull Your Potential, by W. Timothy Gallwey. Renowned sports psychology expert W. Timothy Gallwey teams up with two esteemed physicians to offer a unique and empowering guide to mental health in today's volatile world. *The Inner Game of Stress* applies the trusted principles of Gallwey's wildly popular Inner Game series, which have helped athletes the world over, to the management of everyday stress—personal, professional, financial, physical—and shows us how to access our inner resources to maintain stability and achieve success.

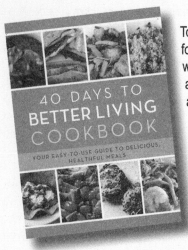